Fast Facts About PTSD: A Guide for Nurses a

Fast Facts for the NEW NURSE PRACTITIONE. Edition (*Aktan*)

Fast Facts for the ER NURSE: Emergency Department Orientation in a Nutshell, Third Edition (*Buettner*)

Fast Facts About GI AND LIVER DISEASES FOR NURSES: What APRNs Need to Know in a Nutshell (*Chaney*)

Fast Facts for the MEDICAL–SURGICAL NURSE: Clinical Orientation in a Nutshell (*Ciocco*)

Fast Facts on COMBATING NURSE BULLYING, INCIVILITY, AND WORKPLACE VIOLENCE: What Nurses Need to Know in a Nutshell (*Ciocco*)

Fast Facts for the NURSE PRECEPTOR: Keys to Providing a Successful Preceptorship in a Nutshell (*Ciocco*)

Fast Facts for the OPERATING ROOM NURSE: An Orientation and Care Guide, Second Edition (*Criscitelli*)

Fast Facts for the ANTEPARTUM AND POSTPARTUM NURSE: A Nursing Orientation and Care Guide in a Nutshell (*Davidson*)

Fast Facts for the NEONATAL NURSE: A Nursing Orientation and Care Guide in a Nutshell (*Davidson*)

Fast Facts Workbook for CARDIAC DYSRHYTHMIAS AND 12-LEAD EKGs (*Desmarais*)

Fast Facts About PRESSURE ULCER CARE FOR NURSES: How to Prevent, Detect, and Resolve Them in a Nutshell (*Dziedzic*)

Fast Facts for the GERONTOLOGY NURSE: A Nursing Care Guide in a Nutshell (*Eliopoulos*)

Fast Facts for the LONG-TERM CARE NURSE: What Nursing Home and Assisted Living Nurses Need to Know in a Nutshell (*Eliopoulos*)

Fast Facts for the CLINICAL NURSE MANAGER: Managing a Changing Workplace in a Nutshell, Second Edition (*Fry*)

Fast Facts for EVIDENCE-BASED PRACTICE IN NURSING: Third Edition (*Godshall*)

Fast Facts for Nurses About HOME INFUSION THERAPY: The Expert's Best Practice Guide in a Nutshell (*Gorski*)

Fast Facts About NURSING AND THE LAW: Law for Nurses in a Nutshell (*Grant, Ballard*)

Fast Facts for the L&D NURSE: Labor & Delivery Orientation in a Nutshell, Second Edition (*Groll*)

Fast Facts for the RADIOLOGY NURSE: An Orientation and Nursing Care Guide in a Nutshell (*Grossman*)

Fast Facts in HEALTH INFORMATICS FOR NURSES (*Hardy*)

Fast Facts on ADOLESCENT HEALTH FOR NURSING AND HEALTH PROFESSIONALS: A Care Guide in a Nutshell (*Herrman*)

Fast Facts for the CRITICAL CARE NURSE, Second Edition (*Hewett*)

Fast Facts for the FAITH COMMUNITY NURSE: Implementing FCN/Parish Nursing in a Nutshell (*Hickman*)

Fast Facts for the CARDIAC SURGERY NURSE: Caring for Cardiac Surgery Patients, Third Edition (*Hodge*)

Fast Facts About the NURSING PROFESSION: Historical Perspectives in a Nutshell (*Hunt*)

Fast Facts for the NURSE PSYCHOTHERAPIST: The Process of Becoming (*Jones, Tusaie*)

Fast Facts for the CLINICAL NURSING INSTRUCTOR: Clinical Teaching in a Nutshell, Third Edition (*Kan, Stabler-Haas*)

Fast Facts for the WOUND CARE NURSE: Practical Wound Management in a Nutshell (*Kifer*)

Fast Facts About EKGs FOR NURSES: The Rules of Identifying EKGs in a Nutshell (*Landrum*)

Fast Facts for the TRAVEL NURSE: Travel Nursing in a Nutshell (*Landrum*)

Fast Facts for the SCHOOL NURSE: What You Need to Know, Third Edition (*Loschiavo*)

Fast Facts to LOVING YOUR RESEARCH PROJECT: A Stress-Free Guide for Novice Researchers in Nursing and Healthcare (*Marshall*)

Fast Facts for MANAGING PATIENTS WITH A PSYCHIATRIC DISORDER: What RNs, NPs, and New Psych Nurses Need to Know (*Marshall*)

Fast Facts About SUBSTANCE USE DISORDERS: What Every Nurse, APRN, and PA Needs to Know (*Marshall, Spencer*)

Fast Facts About CURRICULUM DEVELOPMENT IN NURSING: How to Develop and Evaluate Educational Programs in a Nutshell, Second Edition (*McCoy, Anema*)

Fast Facts for the CATH LAB NURSE (*McCulloch*)

Fast Facts About NEUROCRITICAL CARE: A Quick Reference for the Advanced Practice Provider (*McLaughlin*)

Fast Facts for DNP ROLE DEVELOPMENT: A Career Navigation Guide (*Menonna-Quinn, Tortorella Genova*)

Fast Facts for DEMENTIA CARE: What Nurses Need to Know in a Nutshell (*Miller*)

Fast Facts for HEALTH PROMOTION IN NURSING: Promoting Wellness in a Nutshell (*Miller*)

Fast Facts for STROKE CARE NURSING: An Expert Care Guide, Second Edition (*Morrison*)

Fast Facts for the MEDICAL OFFICE NURSE: What You Really Need to Know in a Nutshell (*Richmeier*)

Fast Facts for the PEDIATRIC NURSE: An Orientation Guide in a Nutshell (*Rupert, Young*)

Fast Facts About FORENSIC NURSING: What You Need to Know (*Scannell*)

Fast Facts About the GYNECOLOGICAL EXAM: A Professional Guide for NPs, PAs, and Midwives, Second Edition (*Secor, Fantasia*)

Fast Facts for the STUDENT NURSE: Nursing Student Success in a Nutshell (*Stabler-Haas*)

Fast Facts About RELIGION FOR NURSES: Implications for Patient Care (*Taylor*)

Fast Facts for CAREER SUCCESS IN NURSING: Making the Most of Mentoring in a Nutshell (*Vance*)

Fast Facts for the TRIAGE NURSE: An Orientation and Care Guide, Second Edition (*Visser, Montejano*)

Fast Facts for DEVELOPING A NURSING ACADEMIC PORTFOLIO: What You Really Need to Know in a Nutshell (*Wittmann-Price*)

Fast Facts for the HOSPICE NURSE: A Concise Guide to End-of-Life Care (*Wright*)

Fast Facts for the CLASSROOM NURSING INSTRUCTOR: Classroom Teaching in a Nutshell (*Yoder-Wise, Kowalski*)

Forthcoming FAST FACTS Books

Fast Facts for NURSE PRACTITIONERS: Current Practice Essentials for the Clinical Subspecialties (*Aktan*)

Fast Facts for the ER NURSE: Guide to a Successful Emergency Department Orientation, Fourth Edition (*Buettner*)

Fast Facts for WRITING THE DNP PROJECT: Effective Structure, Content, and Presentation (*Christenbery*)

Fast Facts for the NURSE PRECEPTOR: Keys to Providing a Successful Preceptorship, Second Edition (*Ciocco*)

Fast Facts for the NEONATAL NURSE: Care Essentials for Normal and High-Risk Neonates, Second Edition (*Davidson*)

Fast Facts About NEUROPATHIC PAIN: What Advanced Practice Nurses and Physician Assistants Need to Know (*Davies*)

Fast Facts about DIVERSITY, EQUITY, AND INCLUSION (*Davis*)

Fast Facts for CREATING A SUCCESSFUL TELEHEALTH SERVICE: A How-to Guide for Nurse Practitioners (*Heidesch*)

Fast Facts for PATIENT SAFETY IN NURSING (*Hunt*)

Fast Facts for DEMENTIA CARE: What Nurses Need to Know, Second Edition (*Miller*)

Fast Facts for NURSE ANESTHESIA (*Moore, Hickman*)

Fast Facts for MAKING THE MOST OF YOUR CAREER IN NURSING (*Redulla*)

Fast Facts for PEDIATRIC PRIMARY CARE: A Guide for Nurse Practitioners and Physician Assistants (*Ruggiero*)

Fast Facts About SEXUALLY TRANSMITTED INFECTIONS (STIs): A Nurse's Guide to Expert Patient Care (*Scannell*)

Fast Facts for the CLINICAL NURSE LEADER (*Wilcox, Deerhake*)

Fast Facts for the HOSPICE NURSE: A Concise Guide to End-of-Life Care, Second Edition (*Wright*)

FAST FACTS for
DNP ROLE DEVELOPMENT

Denise Menonna-Quinn, DNP, RN-BC, AOCNS, BMTCN, began her nursing career as a graduate of the Holy Name Hospital School of Nursing, Teaneck, New Jersey. She always knew she would continue her education with her final goal being a doctoral degree. She graduated from St. Peter's University, Englewood Cliffs, New Jersey, with a bachelor's degree, which was quickly followed by a master's degree in clinical nursing from Seton Hall University, West Orange, New Jersey. She reached her doctoral goal when she completed her doctor of nursing practice (DNP) degree at William Paterson University, Wayne, New Jersey. Dr. Menonna-Quinn is a classroom and clinical instructor at colleges and universities in northern New Jersey, contributing to the education and developing practice of the next generation of nurses. It is her clinical practice where Dr. Menonna-Quinn has made her greatest contributions to nursing. She has dedicated her more than 30-year clinical career to the care of oncology patients in a wide variety of roles, including staff nurse, clinical specialist, breast cancer nurse coordinator, education specialist, insurance nurse navigator for melanoma patients seeking bone marrow transplants, and ambulatory chemotherapy administration nurse. She brings her considerable intellect and passion to the care of complex oncology patients with compassion, resulting in deep and meaningful nurse–patient relationships based on trust and caring.

Toni Tortorella Genova, DNP, APN-C, FNP-BC, NP-C, received her bachelor's degree from SUNY, Downstate College of Nursing, Brooklyn, New York, and her master's degree from the Hunter-Bellevue College of Nursing, New York, New York. Additionally, she received her DNP as a member of the inaugural class of William Paterson University, Wayne, New Jersey, and her post-master's certificate as a family nurse practitioner (FNP) from the University of Massachusetts, Boston, Massachusetts. Dr. Tortorella Genova is a tenured faculty member at Bergen Community College, Paramus, New Jersey. She has 25 years of classroom and clinical teaching experience in medical–surgical nursing. Her role of educator is informed and influenced by her more than 35 years of experience as an oncology nurse in a variety of roles, including staff nurse, manager, clinical nurse specialist, and ambulatory oncology nurse, in multiple hospitals and private practices in the New York-New Jersey metropolitan area. She remains clinically active as a volunteer FNP for a clinic that provides healthcare to the uninsured.

FAST FACTS for
DNP ROLE DEVELOPMENT

A Career Navigation Guide

Denise Menonna-Quinn, DNP, RN-BC, AOCNS, BMTCN
Toni Tortorella Genova, DNP, APN-C, FNP-BC, NP-C

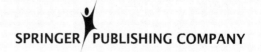

SPRINGER PUBLISHING COMPANY

Springer Publishing Company, LLC
11 West 42nd Street
New York, NY 10036
www.springerpub.com
http://connect.springerpub.com/home

Acquisitions Editor: Adrianne Brigido
Compositor: Amnet Systems

ISBN: 978-0-8261-3684-8
ebook ISBN: 978-0-8261-3685-5
DOI: 10.1891/9780826136855

19 20 21 22 23 / 5 4 3 2 1

Library of Congress Cataloging-in-Publication Data
Names: Menonna-Quinn, Denise, author. | Tortorella Genova, Toni, author.
Title: Fast facts for DNP role development : a career navigation guide /
    Denise Menonna-Quinn, Toni Tortorella Genova.
Other titles: Fast facts (Springer Publishing Company)
Description: New York, NY : Springer Publishing Company, LLC, [2020] |
    Series: Fast facts | Includes bibliographical references and index. |
Identifiers: LCCN 2019040554 (print) | LCCN 2019040555 (ebook) | ISBN
    9780826136848 (paperback) | ISBN 9780826136855 (ebook)
Subjects: MESH: Advanced Practice Nursing—standards | Nurse's Role |
    Career Choice | Advanced Practice Nursing—education | Education,
    Nursing, Graduate
Classification: LCC RT82 (print) | LCC RT82 (ebook) | NLM WY 128 | DDC
    610.7306/9—dc23
LC record available at https://lccn.loc.gov/2019040554
LC ebook record available at https://lccn.loc.gov/2019040555

Contact us to receive discount rates on bulk purchases.
We can also customize our books to meet your needs.
For more information please contact: sales@springerpub.com

I dedicate this book to my amazing family. My husband, Eddie, whose undying support, encouragement, love, and patience, helped shape this book. To my fabulous children, Evan and Natalie, who are my inspiration. Thank you for your continued love and support. I will miss our time working together at the kitchen table. To my parents, Frances and Joseph Menonna, who taught me to always be the best I can be, obtain the highest educational preparation, and, most importantly, never give up. Lastly, to my precious Lucky and Luna for keeping me company during the late-night writing hours.

I must thank my coauthor, Toni Tortorella Genova. Without her intellect, incredible writing skills, and love, this book would not be possible. Additionally, I need to acknowledge and thank my oncology colleagues at the cancer center where I am employed. Their encouragement and support, especially Gina Lione's, is wholeheartedly appreciated.—Denise Menonna-Quinn

I would like to thank my coauthor, Denise Menonna-Quinn, for suggesting this journey into authorship and taking me along for the ride—it's been an adventure! I would also like to thank my cohort members of the inaugural DNP class of William Paterson University in New Jersey, who provide ongoing support and encouragement. I would like to dedicate this book to my family—my husband, Paul; my three children, Alexandra, Andrew, and Amanda and their significant others, Jerry and Jess, for their unwavering love and support; and my parents, Elaine and Vincent Tortorella, who provided me a loving and supportive foundation in life that allows me to believe in myself and tackle new adventures.—Toni Tortorella Genova

Contents

Contributor

Theresa Moore, DNP, RN-BC, NE-BC, CPHIMS
Retired, Fairleigh Dickinson University

Preface

Choosing the journey to pursue a doctoral degree is an exciting time but can also be an arduous experience. This is especially true if one is unsure of the school, program, requirements, and timeline. We were once DNP students with that same list of unanswered questions and uncertainty of the educational and future career path, which led us to the development of this book. We remember sitting in the first DNP class with a lengthy well-written syllabus, a list of requirements, and feelings of uncertainty about a direction for the ever-present DNP project. However, we knew, and had the unwavering belief, that this was the right choice for a terminal degree for us due to its emphasis on clinical practice and patient outcomes. Fast-forward several years: The experience of obtaining the degree, as well as the knowledge gained during its pursuit, has provided the insight, passion, and drive to write about the DNP degree and role development of those nurses who attain it.

We believed it would be extremely helpful to have a practical guidebook that clearly identified the options available to a nurse with a DNP degree. The goal of *Fast Facts for DNP Role Development* is to provide a current overview of the roles that can be held by DNP-prepared nurses and how to successfully use the degree to enhance an individual's practice choices. It emphasizes the different role options available to nurses pursing the DNP degree, including those who remain at the bedside or the clinic and those who assume leadership and faculty positions.

The first chapter discusses the evolution of the DNP degree, as well as the importance and understanding of the American Association of Colleges of Nursing (AACN) DNP essentials. Chapters 2 and 3 emphasize how to operationalize the DNP essentials by providing examples to clarify understanding and utilization.

Part II identifies the individual roles that nurses with DNP degrees could inhabit and acts as guide for DNP-prepared nurses to identify a career path that will best fit their skill, knowledge, and interest levels. This part also addresses strategies for success in the various roles.

We would like to acknowledge our editor, Adrianne Brigido, for listening, guiding, supporting, and, most importantly, believing in the book concept. We would like to recognize Dr. Brenda Marshall, role model extraordinaire, whom we thank for her drive, passion, knowledge, expertise, and loving support. A huge thank-you to our contributing author, Dr. Terri Moore, for her expertise in nursing informatics. A special thank-you to our fellow colleagues Dr. Kimberly Rivera, Dr. Benjamin Evans, Dr. Sharon Puchalski, and Dr. Campbell-O'Dell for eloquently describing the positive impact of the DNP degree on their lives and careers.

As you embark on your journey to pursue a DNP degree, we hope this book will prove helpful in your pursuit. We also hope you enjoy using this guide as much as we enjoyed writing it. We wish you the best of luck. Have fun, and remember, never give up!

Denise Menonna-Quinn
Toni Tortorella Genova

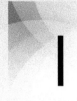

I

The DNP

1

Pursuing the DNP Degree

"For several decades, I had wanted to complete my terminal degree but could not decide on which degree—PhD, EdD, or DNP—as those were the only degrees available for doctoral study at the time. I did not feel called to do bench research or to an academic research degree, so I deferred. With the Institute of Medicine's report On the Future of Nursing, the DNP was initiated. I was invited to attend an information dinner and subsequently was admitted to the first DNP class in New Jersey at the University of Medicine and Dentistry of New Jersey. I completed my degree and earned my DNP. Subsequently, I found that my voice on agency and institutional policies as an administrator began to hold more weight with other disciplines like medicine and pharmacy within the clinical setting, and my expertise and respect in professional and academic circles increased. In the decade since, I've grown as a nursing leader. I have had the honor to serve as an associate vice president for a large medical center, as the first male president for the New Jersey State Nurses Association, and in the role of assistant professor at both state and private universities. Earning my terminal degree in nursing has fulfilled a personal goal that has enriched my life and helped promote my sense of self-worth and integrity. The DNP was the right degree, and I do not regret waiting for its development and availability."—Benjamin Evans, DD, DNP, RN, APN

INTRODUCTION

Overview of the Doctor of Nursing Practice (DNP) Degree

Congratulations! First and foremost, applaud yourself for contemplating, planning, and/or committing to advancing your nursing knowledge and career at the doctorate level. Taking the initial steps toward the most rewarding degree has endless opportunities! So, let us begin and positively leap into pursing, understanding, and maximizing the DNP degree. The DNP is acknowledged as a nursing practice doctorate and has been developed to create expert nurse clinicians regardless of nursing role. The scholarly degree has evolved over the past decade and continues to expand to meet the demand for an increase in the number of doctoral-prepared nurses.

Fast Facts

The DNP degree's focus is based upon current patient healthcare issues, at the levels of the bedside, organization, and community. The DNP degree is a vehicle for nurses to raise awareness of the global nursing aspects and concerns of current health policy and procedures that will ultimately impact patients and their outcomes. Additionally, a primary intent of the DNP degree is to empower nurses to make remarkable changes for patients and organizations within a complex, financially driven, and challenged healthcare system.

For decades, the master of science in nursing (MSN) degree was considered the highest academic degree for clinical nursing professionals, while the PhD was identified as the highest academic degree for nursing researchers. MSN programs have been offered at countless universities around the country. The majority of MSN programs offered students the option to pursue different tracks of practice: nurse practitioner (NP), education, and/or management/leadership. Nurses would have the ability to choose the appropriate path to meet their professional goals and concentrate on track-specific curriculum for their specialty.

However, in the early 2000s, the American Association of Colleges of Nursing (AACN) initiated much discussion and questioned what would be the most favorable terminal/doctoral degree for NPs and clinicians. During the discussions and debates, the AACN nursing leaders were instrumental in the determination of the need for and identification of the nursing practice doctorate—DNP.

TERMINAL DEGREE FOR NURSING

As the healthcare system has become more complex, the need for clinicians to have a broader scope of understanding on how to deliver the highest quality care was identified as a major concern by the nursing profession. It has been noted that clinicians today must be astutely aware of the financial aspects of providing care, including ordering diagnostic tests, prescribing medications, and admitting patients to the hospital. These concerns and challenges in the delivery of care have led to the need for and development of a terminal practice doctoral degree. Therefore, nursing adopted the terminal practice doctorate, which has become the standard for several other healthcare disciplines. The AACN reviewed and researched other clinical specialties, such as physical therapy (DPT), occupational therapy (OTD), pharmacy (PharmD), and audiology (AuD), that have incorporated a practice doctorate as their terminal clinical degree. The nursing practice degree was first introduced as a professional path for NPs to obtain a doctoral practice degree in order to combat the issues of autonomous practice, changing healthcare environment, including the Affordable Healthcare Act, and the shortage of qualified nurse educators. Nursing's ability to utilize the practice doctorate has created a significant increase in the number of nurses pursuing higher education.

In 2006, the terminal degree in nursing dramatically changed with the addition of the DNP. The development and acceptance of the DNP has altered the climate of nursing programs and curricula both nationally and internationally. Canada has been involved in exploring the DNP degree for NPs (Brar, Boschma, & McCuaig, 2010). International nursing schools and universities have been following the progress of the U.S. practice doctorate programs.

In the beginning stages of the development of the DNP program, there existed a significant amount of controversy among the nursing community and nursing scholars. Many nurses questioned the usefulness of the DNP and challenged its creditability. Countless publications in peer-reviewed journal articles highlighted the potential disruption of the practice doctorate. Originally, the DNP degree was specifically aimed to be the highest degree for NPs.

Most DNP programs require the candidate to have an MSN degree, specialty certification and be currently practicing. However, there are some universities that offer a bachelor of science in nursing (BSN) to DNP program embracing the concept that the DNP is a terminal-level degree.

THE USE OF THE "Dr." TITLE

DNP programs have been embraced by the nursing community and recognized as a leader in scholarly nursing practice. Historically, the "Dr." title has evolved from the academic arena since the Middle Ages. The recognition of the DNP as a terminal practice degree has offered the opportunity to use the official "Dr." title. There are numerous definitions related to the term *doctor*. *Doctor* can be used to refer to a professor holding a terminal degree in the academic setting. *Doctor* can also be used to address healthcare professionals, such as physicians, dentists and/or veterinarians.

In most settings, nurses with a DNP degree are using the "Dr." title with little difficulty. For example, in the academic setting, the use of "Dr." is widely accepted among colleagues, students, and universities. Historically, the title "Dr." was initially formed in the academic arena and has been used since the 1800s. In addition to those in academia, DNP-prepared nurses in administration, education, research, and leadership roles can utilize the title "Dr." without controversy. However, this is not true in the practice setting. Unfortunately, the use of the title by DNPs in clinical practice remains a controversial issue among other healthcare providers.

Interestingly, some states do not allow the use of title "Dr." for clinical-practicing DNP nurses.

Fast Facts

Arizona and Delaware have specific legislation for NPs when using the "Dr." title. The NP is required to clearly state his or her role in the introduction.

Certain healthcare organizations may also have specific requirements and/or restrictions for nurses and NPs utilizing the earned "Dr." title. Therefore, it is important for a DNP to investigate and understand an organization's viewpoint and potential restrictions of the earned "Dr." title before making a decision of employment.

The controversy of using the "Dr." title exists among other healthcare providers, and the major concern expressed is the patient may experience role confusion. The rationale used by the medical community for the disagreement toward nurses using the earned "Dr." title is related to the concern that patients will be confused as to who is the medical physician. However, practice confusion can be avoided by NPs and DNPs using clear and distinct nurse–patient communication. For example, a proper DNP introduction in the practice setting includes "Hello, my name is Dr. Susan Smith. I am your nurse practitioner." It is important to address the title issue before entering the workplace, and DNPs need to be confident and professional in presenting themselves to their colleagues and patients.

ADVANTAGES OF THE DNP DEGREE

The DNP degree is a huge accomplishment for the nursing profession. The literature supports that nurses with doctoral degrees account for approximately 1% to 2% of the nursing population. Doctoral degrees included in the literature encompass DNPs, PhDs, and EdDs as well. Statistically, this is a small number of nurses pursuing an advanced degree. However, DNP program enrollment and completion is surpassing that of the PhD programs and continues to increase steadily. Being the DNP is clinically and practice focused, it has afforded nurses across all nursing fields to follow the path of doctoral education. The DNP allows nurses the opportunity, time, resources, and interest to pursue a higher level of education. According to the AACN, currently there are close to 350 DNP programs in the 50 states plus the District of Columbia. There are approximately 121 new DNP programs in the planning stages within the United States. The number of DNP student enrollment from 2017 to 2018 significantly increased from 29,093 to 32,678 (AACN, 2019). This growth indicates the wide acceptance of the DNP degree among the nursing population as a viable option for practice. These numbers speak volumes in the nursing arena. DNP programs provide multiple options for nurses to pursue a terminal degree in nursing. Most importantly, the DNP degree is not isolated to NPs as originally suggested but for all nurses planning to pursue the highest educational experience.

The healthcare environment is multifaceted and requires nurses to have a keen understanding of evidence-based practice/research, health policy, change theories, science of nursing, nursing theories, and business concepts. In order to execute the above mentioned concepts, advanced educational preparation must be the target for nurses and NPs. To deliver high-quality patient outcomes, meet national safety benchmarks, become actively involved with healthcare policy, and maintain a financial balance, a doctorate degree is essential.

Fast Facts

A primary goal for the Institute of Medicine (2010) is the need to double the number of doctoral-prepared nurses by 2020. DNP programs and DNP nurses can be instrumental in reaching the goal.

EVOLUTION OF THE DNP DEGREE

Nursing is a unique profession regarding educational preparation, credentials, and titles. The global changes in healthcare have been a primary reason for the lack of uniformity within educational levels in nursing. For example, a nurse can be eligible for applying to the nursing licensing exam by attending either a diploma, an associate's, or a bachelor's program. There is no standardization of an educational program to become a registered nurse, unlike other healthcare professionals. The reason for the diversity within the educational preparation is directly related to nursing's flexibility. The strategic implementation of numerous options for entering nursing schools was in direct response to the ever-changing global healthcare and patient needs. Nursing created the educational variations and changes to the professional preparation and titles to ensure an opportunity to increase the number of nurses entering the profession and ultimately meeting the demands to care for increased aging patient populations. Examples of how the nursing profession adapted to the changing healthcare environment were the development of licensed practical nurse (LPN) and associate degree (2-year community-based) nursing programs during the times of severe nursing shortages.

Fast Facts

The lack of standardization within nursing has created an alphabet soup of credentials, which has caused discord within the profession and confusion in the healthcare community.

In some instances, it has led to a lack of respect for nursing among other healthcare professionals, as nursing does not follow a uniform approach to the educational preparation. The AACN needs to be recognized as a leader and motivator for the nursing profession. The DNP degree should be viewed as a vehicle and innovator for nurses to obtain a terminal degree. The DNP degree has highlighted a clinical practice doctorate and has empowered nurses and NPs. DNP nurses have the ability to directly impact the perception of the nursing profession as well as have an opportunity to provide the highest quality care within a complex healthcare system. NPs and DNPs are leaders within the profession and can be viewed as change agents.

The AACN was at the forefront of the development of the DNP degree. The concept originated from the AACN in 2002. A task force was formed to determine and answer the question regarding a practice doctorate. Although a practice doctoral degree was not a new idea, the ability to successfully implement a standardized practice program was not yet established. In addition, complete endorsement of the practice degree was not widely accepted.

In 1979, the Frances Payne Bolton School of Nursing was the leader and first to create a DNP program. The program was based upon the enhancement of clinical expertise and expansion of education through leadership and research.

Source: Frances Payne Bolton School of Nursing. (n.d.). *Doctor of nursing practice*. Retrieved from https://case.edu/nursing/programs/dnp

In order for the practice degree to come to life, the AACN task force worked diligently on reviewing the preexisting practice programs, determining the purpose of the degree, initiating appropriate terminology/verbiage goals, and proposing a path for curriculum development. In 2004, the AACN published a position statement, which clearly outlined the benefits of the practice doctorate, and hence, the adoption of the DNP as the terminal practice degree became illuminated. The position paper emphasized that the DNP program must develop advanced competencies for complicated health practice and faculty members; pursue leadership roles; impact nursing practice and patient outcomes; strengthen care delivery; provide advanced practice knowledge without a strong research component; improve program requirements, credits, time, and credentials; provide a venue to attract nonnursing individuals to the profession; and ultimately increase faculty to provide clinical instruction.

After the decision to proceed with the practice degree, the AACN initiated another task force. This time, the task force was assigned the mission of developing the requirements and expectations of the degree. The major component of the task force was the establishment of the DNP essentials (AACN, 2006). These essentials serve as the foundation of the degree and act as a guide to mold the curricula and programs that are currently in existence.

NURSING ROLES FOR THE DNP DEGREE

As previously mentioned, the DNP was specifically designed as the entry-level degree for the NP and has evolved to include nurses practicing in direct patient care or indirect patient care roles. The ability for nurses to apply to DNP programs regardless of their specialty or nursing role contributes to the successful growth of these programs. Nurses are expanding their educational process because of the desire for advanced knowledge, practice, competencies, theories, evidence-based practice, and research.

Direct patient care is associated with the hands-on approach encompassing inpatient or outpatient settings, ED, critical care, oncology, cardiology, and medical/surgical nursing, to name a few examples. The advanced nursing roles such as NP and clinical nurse specialists also qualify as direct patient care. The role of DNP direct care provider is focused around the patient and family. It is imperative for the DNP provider to review and understand the patient's disease process and pay special attention to critical labs, diagnostic tests, and current treatment options in order to implement and ensure positive clinical outcomes. The DNP emphasis is to provide high-quality outcomes for patients and their family members.

The roles of indirect nursing incorporate management/leadership and education. Indirect nursing roles influence the patient from a global aspect. Patients are affected by the changes in healthcare from the governmental policies or state-level organizational policy and procedures and identification of educational deficiencies. For example, indirect nursing roles that have correlation to patient care have been the changes in fall policy and procedures, alterations in visitation times for critical care and oncology units, and the development of bloodless medicine centers. The staff development/education DNP role can also impact patient care. For example, the development of new and updated hospital-based educational programs, such as advanced emergency/critical care, oncology/bone marrow transplant, and maternal/child health, will ultimately influence patient care. Some hospitals are on the cutting edge of new nurse orientations and include advanced simulation classes. Regardless of how or where a DNP chooses to practice, the DNP degree will afford the chance to explore the following in depth: difficult patient issues and

12

PART I THE DNP

procedures; controversial, ethically charged patient situations; and
the ability to implement change in any practice setting.

DIFFERENCES IN DOCTORAL PROGRAMS

Diversity is a common theme in nursing. Educational programs are
varied and have different requirements based upon the curriculum and
goal of the degree. As stated previously, there are numerous educational
paths to receive a registered nurse title; now the same holds true for a
doctoral degree. There is no one-size-fits-all in nursing; however, it is
imperative for students to pursue the degree that will match/fit best in
their career goals and lifelong plans. There are three options from which
to choose regarding doctoral degrees: DNP, PhD, and EdD. These are all
considered terminal degrees and can yield multiple options in relation
to the nursing profession. It is important to remember that each degree
has its own distinct feature, which will add to the current nursing arena.

Fast Facts

The DNP is known as a clinical/practice-based degree, the PhD is
primarily a research-based degree, and the EdD has an educational
focus.

One degree is not better than the other. What is most significant
is that the appropriate degree is chosen based upon an individual's
professional and personal long-term career goals. Making a decision to engage in doctoral education should not be taken lightly, and
one should research and investigate several universities and options
before making the final decision.

In some instances, a student may decide to obtain a dual doctoral
degree. After reviewing the differences, some may determine that in
order to create a diverse career path, two degrees may be a perfect
match. In some rare instances, a nurse may aspire to be a perpetual
student and enjoy the vigorous thought-provoking stimulation of
learning. In any event, whatever the reason and choice, a doctoral
education is one of the most rewarding experiences. Table 1.1 reviews
the differences between the doctoral degrees.

Table 1.1

	DNP	PhD	EdD
Differences Between the DNP, PhD, and EdD Degrees			
Fundamentals of the degree	Practice/clinical based or focused	Research focused	Education focused
	Clinical practice, leadership, education, and not limited to nurse practitioners	Nursing theory	Learning and teaching theories and strategies
			Solving problems in educational systems
			Research concepts
Goals	Translation of a research expert in a clinical field	Development of research in specific specialty in nursing	Development of sound nursing educational programs (including at the classroom and organizational levels)
Prerequisites (highly dependent on each individual college/university)	MSN or BSN degree (some schools will offer a BSN to DNP, which requires more credit hours)	Usually MSN (some schools will accept BSN candidates)	Master's degree in related field
			Relevant work experiences
Each requires letters of recommendation	**Some programs may require current certification in related specialty**		
Average credit hours	70–90 with BSN to DNP	60 credit hours, including dissertation hours	60 credit hours
Part-time and full-time options	40–50 with MSN to DNP		
Learning methods	In-class	In-class	In-class
Many programs can be offered completely online	Online	Online	Online
	Hybrid courses	Hybrid courses	Hybrid courses

(*continued*)

Table 1.1

Differences Between the DNP, PhD, and EdD Degrees (*continued*)

	DNP	PhD	EdD
Clinical work requirements	A maximum of 1,000 may be required by some programs	Minimal clinical hours are usually required	May require workshops, research in the community, and classroom time and evaluation
Research requirements	Statistics Research concepts Nursing and change theory	Extensive faculty-guided research in related specialty	Research concepts with educational focus
Final project requirements	Final project may consist of a form of evidence-based project, performance improvement, quality-driven project, presentation, and/or published scholarly paper	Research-based dissertation in the specialty of nursing	Cumulative project, research, and scholarly publication in related specialty
Career opportunities	Clinical practice Leadership roles Academic roles (may have challenges in pursuing tenured track programs) Health policy roles	Academic roles (tenured track) Nurse researcher	Academic roles (tenured track) Professional development Private organizational education

FINANCIAL CONSIDERATIONS FOR THE DNP DEGREE

Finances may be a concern in pursuing a doctoral degree. However, there are several resources that need to be explored before making money a barrier to achieving one's goal. DNP students working full time in healthcare organizations may have the advantage of tuition reimbursement. If tuition reimbursement is available, make sure to read the policy and deadline dates. Some organizations require final grades for courses to be registered in a computerized system or directly communicated to the human resources department by a specific date and time in order to be eligible for the reimbursement. Grades may also be another factor in the eligibility for tuition assistance, and most often the requirement is a C or better. However, maintaining adequate grades in the program is less likely to be a problem for DNP students compared with undergraduate and graduate students. Typically, doctoral students are highly motivated, extremely bright, and eager to learn.

Scholarships and grants are other viable options for tuition assistance. It is a crucial factor to remain diligent and pay special attention to requirements and deadlines when engaging in scholarships and grant applications. Some applications may require letters of recommendation; therefore, it is imperative to allot adequate time to make the request to fellow colleagues and provide them a specific deadline.

Specialty organizations usually offer scholarship opportunities at annual conferences and to the members of the organization. Therefore, being a member can yield numerous benefits. It is important to review the requirements and submit by the deadlines. Applying for scholarships and grants may take time and coordination; however, the results can be quite lucrative. Scholarships can range from $1,000 to $2,500. In some cases, scholarly grants, which usually require a significant amount of information, can be awarded from $10,000 to $60,000, depending on the topic and potential anticipated outcomes. Some faculty members may be able to assist in the process of grant writing if the topic is appropriate. Individual scholarships can be another option, such as from local businesses, community groups, and private corporations; these often provide a small sum of money, but it is worth completing the application process.

Lastly, scholarship and work study programs at the university/ college level can be offered to students. These are usually limited, are highly competitive, and require a separate application process. Students are usually selected based upon the program chair and have to meet specific criteria. Additionally, some programs offer a stipend for graduate students who work with faculty on individual projects not related to the DNP project and may be required to work 10 to

20 hours per week. The amount of work time required is dependent on the program and the available resources. It is important to connect with the dean or program director regarding scholarships and work programs to gain information and access to the application process.

VARIETY OF DNP PROGRAMS

Just like there are no two nurses, patients, families, and physicians who are exactly the same, the same holds true for DNP programs. The AACN developed key elements, including the competencies of the DNP essentials; however, each curriculum is significantly different. DNP curricula are built upon the foundation of traditional master's programs that are highly focused on utilizing evidence-based practice, quality improvement, patient outcomes, leadership skills, and organizational systems concepts. It is important to understand that DNP programs may include specific aspects of research methods and theories, which can be incorporated into the final project.

The majority of the DNP programs will offer different teaching styles/methods, which include either face-to-face or online interactions or a combination of the two strategies. Some universities have named their programs "hybrid classroom learning." Regardless of the terminology used by the university or college to implement the DNP program, the most important decision is that a student makes the right choice for his or her learning needs, work requirements, and lifestyle.

DNP program educators are cognizant that DNP students are often working part time or full time. Many times, DNP programs encourage DNP students to continue to stay involved with patient care, as this is a practice doctorate and allows students to remain current in their area of expertise. DNP programs may utilize mixed teaching methodology, such as in-person class time, which may often be scheduled on weekends and/or designated times during the semester. Another variation of class time is to have students attend extended time on campus at the beginning or end of the semester and the rest of the time use distance-learning concepts. Lastly, there are many DNP programs that are purely online. Online courses are organized to include required assignments and specific deadlines and are presented at the beginning of the course. The opportunities are endless and offer multiple avenues to be successful in pursuing a DNP degree.

DNP students need to understand their learning styles to find the best match and to strike a healthy balance between work and school.

Fast Facts

It is highly suggested to write a list of pros and cons of different programs and take into account which will offer the best chance of completing the degree. The goal is to align the professional and personal goals with that of the university.

Numerous DNP programs use the concept of educational nursing cohorts. A "cohort" is a group of students who are educated at the same time with a specific curriculum. There are many advantages of cohorts, and they have been used primarily for higher education. A nursing cohort is beneficial to DNP students because it provides small group dynamics; fosters support, teamwork, and collaboration; and utilizes each student's individual strengths, which create an environment to share resources. Additionally, nursing cohorts open perspectives on other nursing specialty areas. For example, members in a nursing cohort can be from different practice settings, such as oncology, administration, maternal–fetal medicine, and informatics, to name a few. Each nurse will bring a wealth of knowledge related to his or her expertise. The ability to share patient experiences, current practice methods, concerns, and barriers creates a chance to eliminate silos among nurses' specialties. In some instances, nurses may recognize that each specialty may encounter similar challenges and/or outcomes within different patient populations. Sharing of knowledge enhances the respect for how other disciplines practice and provides a network of resources that can be used after completing the DNP degree. Nursing cohorts also create positive bonds between the members and can be the foundation for lifelong friendships and collaboration.

REQUIREMENTS FOR DNP PROGRAMS

A universal requirement of DNP programs is the completion of clinical hours. Some programs can require as much as 1,000 clinical hours. Depending upon the university and curriculum design, there are a variety of mechanisms to reach the 1,000 hours. Some courses may have embedded clinical hours, whereas others are correlated with the DNP project. The amount of clinical hours is also dependent on the degree while entering the DNP program. For example, those who have a BSN degree may require more clinical hours than a nurse entering with an MSN degree. The dean or program director will be able to assist with questions and concerns regarding meeting the clinical requirements.

Perseverance, dedication, positivity, hard work, and time management are all skills required to fulfill the DNP program requirements. Time management is truly the key to success and will allow the ability to envision the end result, the final project. Words cannot describe the thrill and elation walking on stage or across the stadium at the respective university and being announced as doctor of nursing practice.

THE DNP PROJECT

The DNP project is the pinnacle for completion of the degree. Much like the nursing profession, there is not a standardized terminology for the project. Each program will identify the project by a different name or title. This is an excellent example of semantics; however, it really does not matter what the final project is named. What matters is that it meets the requirements of the curriculum and that it is scholarly based and completed within the allotted time. Common terms for the DNP project include *capstone, DNP project, final project, evidence-based project, quality improvement,* and *scholarly project.* The project is designed to identify challenges in healthcare, current issues in the practice setting, and health policy concerns. The results of the project are to ultimately provide a potential solution, strategy, and/or increased awareness and understanding of the potential issue. Additionally, the project is to add to the body of knowledge and nursing literature.

Another factor regarding the DNP project is the potential influences of the teaching faculty. For example, if the faculty member is teaching with a PhD background, the project may be based on a more traditional research approach. Conversely, if a DNP faculty is teaching, the focus may be on a single evidence-based project, a quality improvement issue on a nursing unit, community health issue, or a current health policy concern. For example, DNP projects range from students developing a preop and postop checklist, to performing a meta-analysis of the role of the DNP, to determining the usage of personal protective equipment among oncology nurses. There is a great deal of diversity among the DNP projects. Each project adds to the nursing knowledge and expertise within the specialty. More importantly, it provides value to the DNP degree, and in certain instances, it can be the beginning of further study. Therefore, one project is not better than another, and what matters the most is that the project is special to the individual practice. Regardless of what the project is named or termed, it is imperative to have careful consideration of the topic before final decision.

The curriculum will dictate the specific requirements for the DNP project but most will include a well-thought-out question, a comprehensive review of the literature, use of tool (if applicable), connection to essentials, plan of implementation, review of data collection, analysis of the outcomes, relationship to nursing practice, and conclusion. In order to avoid struggling with project selection, choose a topic that sparks passion and one that will have the ability to develop a deep connection with and impact individual practice. The DNP essentials will be another factor in topic selection. The essentials will assist in narrowing the focus of the project and, once incorporated, will guide the method and outcomes to final results.

The DNP project will be infused into daily life for a brief period of time. Remember there is a beginning and an end to the DNP project. Just before the completion of the project, it may take on a life of its own. However, faculty guidance, time management, and endurance will lead to the final product. There may be some days when the project is more important than eating and sleeping! Just know that once final papers are signed, the project will be laid to rest and forever in print. Don't ever give up!

In most programs, a project chairperson will be determined through a proposal committee. During this time, faculty members listen and review the DNP student presentations of the DNP project. The committee helps the student to determine if the project is acceptable, clinically significant, and implementable. Usually, the faculty chairperson and the student will develop a mutual agreement to work together. This is a time for the student to decide who will be the best person to assist and guide him or her through the DNP project. Having a relationship with the chair is paramount in the completion process. The chairperson has an integral role in assisting the student navigate through the project, providing positive and negative feedback, evoking critical thinking, critiquing scholarly writing, and ensuring the student is prepared for oral and written presentation (if applicable).

FUTURE DIRECTIONS: BRIDGE PROGRAMS

Oftentimes, the DNP project can take on a life of its own, requiring further refinement, and can be the foundation of another degree. Please note this path is not for everyone, but for some, the DNP may be the first doctoral degree. For others, the DNP is the pinnacle degree for practice and needs no further education. As this is a controversial issue, the goal of this book is to provide all options that may or may not be a choice of the reader. Bridge programs exist and may be a viable option for those who have been ignited from their work in their DNP program and want to delve deeper into the research focus. Many students may be sparked and motivated to add to the educational repertoire.

In contrast, this may sound overwhelming at this point in time because many are still deciding or planning on completing the DNP degree. However, it is important to think ahead toward the future in order to align yourself in the best possible position to navigate through your educational and professional journey. The objective is to increase awareness of the vast opportunities that can be built upon the DNP degree.

The DNP affords the best degree for practice nurses; however, if you decide to add upon the practice aspect and pursue research and or academia, a dual doctorate may be a viable consideration. A bridge program may offer a chance to obtain a dual doctorate with either a PhD or an EdD, depending on which nursing role you chose to practice. When deciding to further your doctoral education, make sure that you choose the best program that will match with your career goals.

Fast Facts

When investigating a bridge program, look for programs that link DNP to PhD or DNP to EdD. The DNP role will prepare you to adequately research the credit requirements, timeline of completion, financial impact, location, and, most importantly, time required on campus.

Some universities will provide a "bridge program" that will accept approximately half of the credits based upon the DNP program. However, not all programs will accept DNP credits; so be careful in university selection. It would be advisable to take the time and call/email the program coordinator.

Some programs will request informal transcripts at first in order to determine how many credits of the DNP will be accepted or require informal transcripts to initiate the application process. Often times, the application process for doctoral degrees have rolling admission and do not have hard stop deadlines.

POSITIVE IMPACT OF THE DNP DEGREE

The DNP is a practice doctorate degree that focuses on the importance of patients' outcomes and the existing difficult and unanswered healthcare dilemmas. The DNP incorporates the elements of nursing theories; understands patient care issues; and reviews current healthcare agendas, policies, and procedures, while utilizing the scholarly thinking and writing process. The DNP degree will allow the nurse to investigate and understand evidence-based practice, research, performance improvement, and quality concerns. The degree will cultivate academic/professional writing, which will be a welcomed addition to the nursing literature.

Obtaining the DNP degree will broaden views regarding all aspects of nursing as well as allow the opportunity to apply strategies and changes to each nursing setting and specialty. On a professional level, the DNP degree will enhance critical/global thinking, which will have the capacity to resonate to patients and organizations.

On the personal level, completing the DNP degree will provide enormous growth and satisfaction. A major accolade for the DNP degree is that it has the capability to be tailored to match individual strengths and professional and personal interests, and most importantly, it will be the fuel for long-term career goals. The achievement of the DNP degree will not only be professionally and personally rewarding but add to current nursing literature and knowledge and allow the prospect to become actively involved in creating nursing history. The DNP opportunities are boundless and will build upon the fundamentals of nursing practice.

SUMMARY

This chapter provided an overview of the evolution of the DNP degree, different programs, and learning environments available. In addition, it is hoped that this chapter will create a vision for potential personal and professional options offered with pursing the degree. Choosing the DNP degree will enhance multiple opportunities to open pathways in nursing that are not always available without a terminal degree.

REFLECTION QUESTIONS

1. What factors influenced your decision to pursue a DNP degree?
2. If you were a chosen member of the AACN task force in 2004, is there any aspect of the position paper that you would have added or deleted in regards to the development of the DNP degree?
3. What are your feelings/concerns about using the title "Dr." in clinical practice?
4. On what nursing specialty do you plan to focus in your DNP project?
5. What change in practice do you envision your DNP project to accomplish?

References

American Association of Colleges of Nursing. (2004). *AACN position statement on the practice doctorate in nursing.* Retrieved from https://www.aacnnursing.org/Portals/42/News/Position-Statements/DNP.pdf

American Association of Colleges of Nursing. (2006). *The essential of doctoral education for advanced nursing practice.* Retrieved from https://www.aacnnursing.org/Portals/42/Publications/DNPEssentials.pdf

American Association of Colleges of Nursing. (2019). *Fact sheet: The doctor of nursing practice (DNP).* Retrieved from https://www.aacnnursing.org/Portals/42/News/Factsheets/DNP-Factsheet.pdf

Brar, K., Boschma, G., & McCuaig, F. (2010). The development of nurse practitioner preparation beyond the master's level: What is the debate about? *International Journal of Nurse Education Scholarship, 7.* doi:10.2202/1548-923X.1928

Frances Payne Bolton School of Nursing. (n.d.). Doctor of nursing practice. Retrieved from https://case.edu/nursing/programs/dnp

Institute of Medicine. (2010). *The future of nursing: Leading change, advancing health.* Washington, DC: National Academies Press. Retrieved from https://www.ncbi.nlm.nih.gov/books/NBK209880/

Further Reading

Dols, J., Hernández, C., & Miles, H. (2017). The DNP project: Quandaries for nursing scholars. *Nursing Outlook, 65,* 84–93. doi:10.1016/j.outlook.2016.07.009

Fredriksson, J. J., Mazzocato, P., Muhammed, R., & Savage, C. (2017). Business model framework applications in health care: A systematic review. *Health Services Management Research, 30,* 219–226. doi:10.1177/0951484817726918

Nurse Journal (n.d.). Financial aid overview and scholarship. Retrieved from https://nursejournal.org/articles/nursing-scholarships-grants

Nurse Practitioner Schools. (n.d.). DNP vs PhD in nursing: What's the difference? Retrieved https://www.nursepractitionerschools.com/faq/difference-between-dnp-phd-nursing

Redman, R., Pressler, S., Furspan, P., & Potempa, K. (2015). Nurses in the United States with a practice doctorate: Implication for leading in the current context of health care. *Nursing Outlook, 63,* 124–129. doi:10.1016/j.outlook.2014.08.003

Smeltzer, S., Sharts-Hopko, N., Cantrell, M., Heverly, M., Nthenge S., & Jenkinson, A. (2015). A profile of US nursing faculty in research and practice-focused doctoral education. *Journal of Nursing Scholarship, 47,* 178–185. doi:10.1111/jnu.12123

Vanderbilt University School of Nursing. (2018). *Curriculum.* Retrieved from https://nursing.vanderbilt.edu/dnp/dnp_curriculum.php

2

Making Sense of the DNP Essentials

"The DNP degree has allowed my career to move from the junior leagues to a world-class opportunity to impact healthcare outcomes. Being a part of the DNP community has opened windows to talented colleagues, evolving healthcare systems, and progressive academic initiatives. Collectively, we are growing our nursing profession to influence the trajectory of healthcare services. This degree has been an opportunity of a lifetime. If you are considering this degree, or if you are already in DNP-prepared practice, enjoy the synergy of talent and focus to assure collective success by improving healthcare outcomes."
—David G. Campbell-O'Dell, DNP, APRN, FNP-BC, FAANP

INTRODUCTION

The DNP Essentials

The doctor of nursing practice (DNP) Essentials are the outline for curriculum design and development of the DNP degree. The DNP Essentials must be present in the DNP programs. An important factor to understand is that each essential was not designed to become a dedicated DNP course. The educators and curriculum designers at the university are responsible for deciding which course will address one individual Essential or multiple Essentials.

The eight Essentials are the foundation of the DNP degree. The American Association of Colleges of Nursing (AACN, 2006) developed the DNP Essentials to act as core competencies for curriculum development in advanced practice roles. The DNP degree fosters numerous roles for nurses in advanced practice capacity as well as individual specialties. The DNP role that a student decides to pursue, such as nurse practitioner, educator, or administrator, will determine the Essential or Essentials on which to concentrate and incorporate into the DNP project.

Fast Facts

The DNP Essentials were developed to broadly be a guide for the development of individual DNP capstone projects.

It is important to make the connection between two or three Essentials in order to create a well-written, organized, and meaningful DNP project. Choosing the appropriate Essentials will aid in the planning, implementation, and development of outcomes for the project. Box 2.1 outlines the eight DNP Essentials.

BOX 2.1 THE EIGHT DNP ESSENTIALS

1. Scientific Underpinnings for Practice
2. Organizational and Systems Leadership for Quality Improvement and Systems Thinking
3. Clinical Scholarship and Analytical Methods for Evidence-Based Practice
4. Information Systems/Technology and Patient Care Technology for the Improvement and Transformation of Health Care
5. Health Care Policy for Advocacy in Health Care
6. Interprofessional Collaboration for Improving Patient and Population Health Outcomes

(continued)

BOX 2.1   THE EIGHT DNP ESSENTIALS *(continued)*

7. Clinical Prevention and Population Health for Improving the Nation's Health
8. Advanced Nursing Practice

Source: American Association of Colleges of Nursing (2006). *The essentials of doctoral education for advanced nursing practice*. Retrieved from https://www .aacnnursing.org/Portals/42/Publications/DNPEssentials.pdf

THE ROLE OF THE ESSENTIALS IN THE DNP CURRICULUM

The Essentials are incorporated into DNP curricula. Some programs will offer a course on a specific Essential, while others may blend several of the Essentials into one course. Each university can approach the presentation of the Essentials in a different fashion. For example, a DNP course entitled Population Health may incorporate other Essentials such as Health Care Advocacy and Inter-Professional Relationship Collaboration for Improving Patient and Population Health Outcomes into the discussions and assignments. Each DNP program has the academic freedom to utilize the Essentials and design the course in a unique way in order to meet the vision and mission of the university. Table 2.1 exhibits examples of DNP course titles and their corresponding DNP Essentials. These titles are from numerous accredited universities within the United States that offer a DNP degree.

Table 2.1

Examples of DNP Course Titles and Corresponding Essentials	
Examples of DNP Course Title in the United States	**Potential Corresponding DNP Essential**
Policy Health Course	Essentials V and VII
Clinical Practicum for Advanced Nursing Practice	Essentials I, VI, and VIII
Transforming the Nation's Health	Essentials IV, VI, and VII
Effective Leadership	Essentials I, II, III, IV, and VI

(continued)

Table 2.1

Examples of DNP Course Titles and Corresponding Essentials (*continued*)

Examples of DNP Course Title in the United States	Potential Corresponding DNP Essential
Scientific Foundations Course	All the essentials may apply
Transformation of Health Care Systems	All the essentials may apply
Informatics for Scholarly Practice	Essentials II, III, IV, and VI
Evidence-Based Practice I and II (*several universities have used these titles*)	Essentials I and III
Management of Organizations and Systems	Essentials I, II, VI, VII and VIII

USING THE DNP ESSENTIALS FOR THE DNP PROJECT

It is vital to have an in-depth understanding of the Essentials in order to create a well-planned, organized, and successful DNP project. The Essentials will have the ability to guide and support the development of the vision of the DNP project.

Fast Facts

The Essentials help guide the appropriate project title, select data collection methods, perform data analysis, and deliver outcomes of the DNP project. Therefore, finding the connection between the Essentials and choosing the most appropriate Essential for the project is imperative and will make the process of completion easier.

Examples of DNP Essentials Used in DNP Projects

Student One: Oncology DNP Project

Student One chose Essentials I (Scientific Underpinnings for Practice) and V (Health Care Policy) for the DNP project that examined the use of personal protective equipment among oncology nurses.

Essential I (Scientific Underpinnings for Practice) describes "actions and advanced strategies to enhance, alleviate, and ameliorate health and healthcare delivery phenomena as appropriate; and evaluate outcomes" (AACN, 2006). The oncology DNP project examined the usage of personal protective equipment between the inpatient and outpatient in a large medical center. Personal protective equipment has been noted as a leading factor in safe handling of chemotherapy agents. Chemotherapy safety measures are behaviors that are fundamental to eliminate or decrease toxic exposure for nurses. Essential I was an excellent choice for this study as it was related to patient and nurse safety, which revolves around practice and quality care measures.

"Health care policy [Essential V]—whether it is created through governmental actions, institutional decision making, or organizational standards—creates a framework that can facilitate or impede the delivery of health care services or the ability of the provider to engage in practice to address health care needs" (AACN, 2006, p. 13). The oncology DNP project identified that there is not a governing body to enforce chemotherapy safety guidelines. The guidelines and recommendations are deferred to be interpreted by individual organizations via their individual policy and procedure manuals. In February 2016, the U.S. Parmacopeial (USP) Convention (2016) published the Chapter 800 Hazardous Drugs Handling in Healthcare Settings, and this year, the USP Convention will be implementing the first government mandate for healthcare providers and organizations to ensure that safety mechanisms are instituted and implemented. The mandate was timely for this student's DNP project, therefore, making Essential V a perfect match (Menonna-Quinn, 2017).

Student Two: Medical/Surgical Pain DNP Project

Student Two explored the medical surgical nurse's knowledge and attitudes regarding pain using a descriptive comparative analysis. This project addressed Essentials I (Scientific Underpinnings for Practice) and III (Clinical Scholarship and Analytical Methods for Evidence-Based Practice).

Essential I delineates the role of the DNP in utilizing knowledge from other disciplines in conjunction with nursing science to provide the highest level of practice to patients. The DNP utilizes a multidisciplinary approach (scientific approach) in identifying healthcare issues and the strategies that can be used to address them efficiently. Scientific theories from nursing and other disciplines are used by the DNP to develop and evaluate new approaches to care and validate those care strategies currently in use. Therefore, Essential I was the driving force for this DNP project. Nurses' knowledge and attitudes regarding pain over a span of 15 years were compared to evaluate whether changes had occurred in this area of patient care. The incorporation of scientific knowledge from the social science to address a patient care issue in nursing meets the demands of Essential I.

Essential III delineates the role of the DNP in the utilization of clinical scholarship and analytical methods for evidence-based practice (EBP). This essential addressed the use of research as a tool for the prepared DNP nurse to develop and evaluate the best evidence for nursing practice and patient-centered issues. The DNP project sought to evaluate whether a change in nurses' knowledge and attitudes regarding pain had occurred over a time period of approximately 15 years. Essential III was the best choice for this project because it allowed the opportunity to use the formal research process beginning with the review of current literature. The methodology was then designed, data were collected and analyzed, outcomes were evaluated, and gaps in practice were identified (Tortorella-Genova, 2014).

Interpretation is a key factor in determining which Essential is the best fit for the DNP project. It is interesting to see how two different DNP projects can use the same Essential and correlate to diverse subject matter. These projects used Essential I from two unique points of view and yet were able to reach the goal of using the Essential to navigate through the planning, implementation, and completion stages of the DNP project. Each student was also able to incorporate other Essentials to connect to the project that represented each's nursing specialty.

ESSENTIAL I: THE SCIENTIFIC UNDERPINNINGS FOR PRACTICE

What do the scientific underpinnings of practice really mean? Essential I needs to be dissected into two sections. Let us begin with the definition of *scientific*. *Scientific* has been defined as utilizing research and investigation in an organized and specific manner. *Underpinning* can be described as the basis and/or foundation of a subject. Combination of the two words makes Essential I an exceptional choice for prepared DNP nurses to identify patient care, clinical assessment, and ethical issues and concerns for the foundation of a project.

Fast Facts

Essential I can incorporate the use of science, nursing, and other theories to explore new concepts and approaches to solve difficult healthcare issues.

DNP Project Topics for Essential I

1. Clinical Patient Care Situations
2. Nurse–Patient Relationships
3. Clinical Treatment Options
4. Assessment Concerns
5. Ethical Situations

ESSENTIAL II: ORGANIZATIONAL AND SYSTEMS LEADERSHIP

Healthcare has significantly changed within the last decade. One of the major changes is the movement of patient-centered care. In this model of delivering care, the patient is the primary focus. The patient's desired healthcare needs are the motivating factors to the decision-making process of treatment options and care. In addition, patient-centered care is customized and collaborative, which means that the patient has an active role in how and what care is delivered. The shift to patient-centered care has impacted organizations' infrastructures and finances. For example, organizations remodeled maternity suites to create an individual soothing home-birthing experience in order to foster family bonding ("What is Patient-Centered Care," 2017.)

Organizations are faced with the need to increase patient satisfaction scores, decrease the use of resources and costs, while at the same time increasing revenue. In order to meet the high demands of the changing healthcare environment, many organizations have adopted the customer-based service model. Patients are now viewed as customers and an active part of the healthcare team.

Fredriksson, Mazzocato, Muhammed, and Savage (2017) conducted a systematic literature review to explain how business model frameworks have been applied to healthcare. The authors found a large increase in business model framework applications over the past decade.

The DNP degree was designed to help meet the changing healthcare demands. The DNP degree has clearly embraced the changes and has developed strategies to deliver advanced high-quality care with the use of the DNP Essentials. Understanding, evaluating, and adjusting healthcare organizational systems are pivotal roles in delivering safe quality patient care within a complex environment.

Fast Facts

Essential II can be used to incorporate quality measures, safety strategies, and communication techniques; identify accountability; and evaluate business plans and leadership decisions, to create a sensitive, safe, caring, and cost-effective health delivery system.

DNP Project Topics for Essential II

1. System Concerns/Failures
2. Medication Administration Situations
3. Leadership/Financial/Business Concerns
4. Evaluation of Individual and Global Policy and Procedures
5. Performance Improvement and Quality Safety Measures

ESSENTIAL III: CLINICAL SCHOLARSHIP AND ANALYTICAL METHODS FOR EBP

The American Association of Colleges of Nursing (2006) elegantly stated "[s]cholarship and research are the hallmarks of doctoral education" (p.11). Nursing has used the knowledge generated from evidence to make significant changes in daily nursing care. EBP can be associated as far back as the days of Florence Nightingale.

Schloman (2001) identified that Florence Nightingale used statistics to explain the multiple causes of death of soldiers during the Crimean War as well as her ability to collect data in an organized/standardized fashion for the army and civilian hospitals. McDonald (2010) also acknowledged Florence's 40 years of applied statistics were used to investigate public healthcare systems. Florence had the forethought to examine maternal mortality during childbirth.

EBP continues to be a vital part of today's nursing process. The DNP project allows for an opportunity to integrate EPB into daily practice and enhance patient outcomes within any nursing specialty. Essential III is associated with the translation of research and its ability to integrate into nursing practice. This Essential combines research methods, such as analytical methods, evaluation and review of current literature, design, data collection, assumptions, analysis of outcomes, and identification of gaps of information as they are related to nursing practice (AACN, 2006).

Fast Facts

Essential III has the flexibility and correlation to be utilized in most DNP projects.

DNP Project Topics for Essential III

1. Evidence-Based Practice Concepts
2. Quality Issues
3. Performance Improvement
4. Patient and Nurse Delivery of Care Concerns
5. Patient and Nurse Research Questions

ESSENTIAL IV: INFORMATION SYSTEMS/TECHNOLOGY AND PATIENT CARE TECHNOLOGY FOR THE IMPROVEMENT AND TRANSFORMATION OF HEALTHCARE

Essential IV is a global topic that encompasses multiple disciplines within the healthcare system. Technology/informatics has been the pinnacle of change in how nurses practice and is the central point for Essential IV. The implementation of electronic medical records (EMRs), medication administration record/system (MAR), and patient access programs have been deemed significant factors in the transformation of care. Filipova (2013) identified that the EMR is a necessary component of information technology. Ajami and Bagheri-Tadi (2013) described the EMR as a critical tool for improving both safety and quality of healthcare.

Moving away from pen and paper has its advantages and disadvantages. Computerized physician order entry (CPOE) can eliminate the risk for translation errors related to medications, but not always 100% of the time. Recent studies have determined that CPOE can still produce medication errors (Korb-Savoldelli, Boussadi, Durieux, & Saatier, 2018; Rouayroux, Calmels, Bachelet, Sallerin, & Divol, 2019). Therefore, technology is both a friend and foe. The DNP-prepared nurse needs to continue to evaluate the informatics aspects of delivering patient care by creating and implementing capstone projects.

Fast Facts

Essential IV can be the leader in the development of many DNP projects with the ultimate focus to improve safe patient care methods across nursing and other healthcare disciplines.

DNP Project Topics for Essential IV

1. Informatics Situations
2. Legal and Ethical Situations
3. Medication Administration Issues
4. Clinical Patient Issues
5. Advances in Medical Devices

ESSENTIAL V: HEALTHCARE POLICY FOR ADVOCACY IN HEALTHCARE

Health policy can be a major focus in DNP curricula, and most universities will offer a course related to health policy in some form. The Institute of Medicine (IOM) report brief (2010) stated "nurses should participate in, and sometimes lead, decision making and be engaged in health care reform-related implementation efforts" (p. 3). This comment directly speaks to the DNPs and nurse practitioners as leaders in the health policy journey. DNP-prepared nurses can be influential in educating other nurses to understand the importance and detailed process of becoming actively involved with health policy.

Health policy development, legislative, and lobbying are multi-faceted, multilayered, and lengthy processes. The course of action for health policy change requires extensive research and in-depth knowledge of the subject as well as an understanding of the political process. In addition, a DNP-prepared nurse needs to be diligent and exhibit excellent interpersonal and communication skills in order to navigate through health policy changes.

Fast Facts

Essential V can be embedded into countless DNP projects and can be at the forefront for change at the bedside, organizational, local, and national levels.

DNP Project Topics for Essential V

1. Current Health Policy
2. Health Disparities
3. Patients With Limited Healthcare Options
4. Local and National Healthcare Issues
5. Quality and Safety Mechanisms

ESSENTIAL VI: INTERPROFESSIONAL COLLABORATION FOR IMPROVING PATIENT AND POPULATION HEALTH OUTCOMES

Essential VI concentrates on leadership and collaboration concepts. This Essential acknowledges the abundant layers associated with providing safe, high-quality, and cost-effective care through positive interprofessional relationships. In order to deliver the best quality care, healthcare providers cannot work within silos. Delivery of care is a group effort with each healthcare provider having a special and important role. An important aspect of interprofessional collaboration is that there needs to be clear expectations and mutual respect for the contributions of each provider. For this to occur and for roles to be understood, excellent open and transparent communication is paramount.

Leading, whether in a formal or informal setting, is hard work. Attributes and key characteristics of good leaders are to be truthful, transparent, understanding, kind, and fair. DNP-prepared nurses can lead at the unit, organizational, and system levels.

Fast Facts

Essential VI can be influential in promoting interprofessional relationships. DNP projects can utilize this Essential to highlight leadership, collaboration, professionalism, and organizational changes to impact patient care, safety measures, and global healthcare issues.

DNP Project Topics for Essential VI

1. Patient Care Issues
2. Difference in Healthcare Practices Among Healthcare Providers
3. Ethical and Organizational Situations
4. Group Dynamics and Communication Techniques
5. Leadership Situation/Concerns

ESSENTIAL VII: CLINICAL PREVENTION AND POPULATION HEALTH FOR IMPROVING THE NATION'S HEALTH

Health promotion is the impetus for Essential VII. The nation is focused on clinical prevention and decreasing unhealthy lifestyles. A national health project is Healthy People 2020, which sets the goals and objectives for 10 years. Healthy People 2020 depicts 42 health topics and approximately 1,200 objectives to improve public health issues (Office of Disease Prevention and Health Promotion [ODPHP], n.d.-a). According to Healthy People 2020, significant improvements have been made in relation to increased life expectancy at birth as well as decreased death rates from heart disease and strokes (ODPHP, 2019). DNP-prepared nurses can be instrumental in recognizing, evaluating, and implementing changes to enhance the public health concerns.

Fast Facts

Essential VII can be the impetus for DNP projects that can examine health situations across all nursing areas.

DNP Project Topics for Essential VII

1. Health Promotion Concepts
2. Public Health Concerns
3. Alcohol and Drug Programs and Smoking Cessation Programs
4. Underserved Patient Populations
5. Global Health Disparities

ESSENTIAL VIII: ADVANCED PRACTICE NURSING

Specialization is the key component to Essential VIII. There are numerous nursing specialties, and it would be impossible for a DNP-prepared nurse to master each of them. Therefore, Essential VIII was designed to create competences for DNP nurses to master advanced knowledge and expertise in a desired nursing specialty area. The ANCC elegantly stated "this distinctive specialization is a hallmark of the DNP" (p. 16). Essential VIII is focused around the ability for the DNP nurse to have advanced health assessment and critical thinking skills as well as integrate and implement cultural sensitivity within the chosen nursing specialty.

Fast Facts

Essential VIII can be the foundation for several DNP projects by exploring and utilizing the key elements of advanced nursing practice, such as critical thinking, advanced health assessment, cultural sensitivity, and EBP concepts.

DNP Project Topics for Essential VIII

1. Diverse Nursing Specialties
2. Cultural Patient Concerns
3. Patient Assessment and Treatment Issues
4. Mentorship and Leadership Issues
5. EBP Concepts

SUMMARY OF ESSENTIALS

The Essentials are the foundation and guide for the DNP degree as well as the DNP project. Depending on the topic, there may be several Essentials that can best be utilized. Each Essential has a unique and individual focus; however, the Essentials are broad enough to be interpreted to meet the needs of different specialties and roles in advanced nursing. The founders of the DNP had the foresight to create the Essentials, which are now critical to pursue the DNP degree and complete the desired project.

REFLECTION QUESTIONS

1. Reflect on the importance of the DNP Essentials.
2. If you were the curriculum designer at your university/college, which Essentials would you develop into a separate course? And why?
3. Which Essential or Essentials have the most meaning for your daily practice?
4. Reflect on the differences and similarities between Essentials V and VI.
5. Reflect on how Essential IV can impact your organization or practice. What advantages and disadvantages do technology systems lend to your practice?
6. What preventive measures would benefit your specialty area and impact the nation's health plan?

References

Ajami, S., & Bagheri-Tadi, T. (2013). Barriers for adopting electronic health records (EHRs) by physicians. *Acta Informatica Medica, 21*, 129–134. doi:10.5455/aim.2013.21.129-134

American Association of Colleges of Nursing. (2006). *The essential of doctoral education for advanced nursing practice.* Retrieved from https://www.aacnnursing.org/Portals/42/Publications/DNPEssentials.pdf

Filipova, A. (2013). Electronic health records use and barriers and benefits to use in skilled nursing facilities. *Computers, Informatics Nursing, 31*, 305–318. doi:10.1097/NXN.0b013e318295e40e

Fredriksson, J., Mazzocato, P., Muhammed, R., & Savage, C. (2017). Business model framework applications in health care: A systematic review. *Health Services Management Research, 30*, 219–226. doi:10.1177/0951484817726918

Institute of Medicine. (2010). *The future of nursing: Leading change, advancing health* [Report brief]. Retrieved from http://nationalacademies.org/hmd/~/media/Files/Report%20Files/2010/The-Future-of-Nursing/Future%20of%20Nursing%202010%20Report%20Brief.pdf

Korb-Savoldelli, V., Boussadi, A., Durieux, P., & Sabatier, B. (2018). Prevalence of computerized physician order entry systems–related medication prescription errors: A systematic review. *International Journal of Medical Informatics, 111*, 112–122. doi:10.1016/j.ijmedinf.2017.12.022

McDonald, L. (2010). Florence Nightingale: Passionate statistician. *Journal of Holistic Nursing, 28*(1), 92–98. doi:10.1177/0898010109358769

Menonna-Quinn, D. (2017). *Usage of personal protective equipment among oncology nurses* (Unpublished doctoral dissertation). William Paterson University, Wayne, New Jersey.

Office of Disease Prevention and Health Promotion. (n.d.-a). About the data. Retrieved from https://www.healthypeople.gov/2020/data-search/About-the-Data

Office of Disease Prevention and Health Promotion. (2019). Retrieved from https://www.healthypeople.gov/2020/About-Healthy-People

Rouayroux, N., Calmels, V., Bachelet, B., Sallerin, B., & Divol, E. (2019). Medication prescribing errors: A pre -and post-computerized physician order entry retrospective study. *International Journal of Clinical Pharmacy, 41*, 228–236. doi:10.1007/s11096-018-0747-0

Schloman, B. F. (2001). Using health statistics: A Nightingale legacy. *Online Journal of Issues in Nursing, 6*(3), 7. Retrieved from http://ojin.nursingworld.org/MainMenuCategories/ANAMarketplace/ANAPeriodicals/OJIN/TableofContents/Volume62001/No3Sept01/UsingHealthStatistics.html

Scientific. (n.d.). In Merriam-Webster's online dictionary. Retrieved from https://www.merriam-webster.com/dictionary/scientific

Tortorella-Genova, T. (2014). *Evaluating medical-surgical nurses' knowledge and attitudes regarding pain: A descriptive comparative analysis* (Published doctoral dissertation). William Paterson University, Wayne, New Jersey. Retrieved from https://pqdtopen.proquest.com/pubnum/3617158.html

Underpinning. (n.d.). In Merriam-Webster's online dictionary. Retrieved from https://www.merriam-webster.com/dictionary/underpinning

U.S. Parmacopeial Convention. (2016). *800 hazardous drugs—Handling in healthcare settings.* Retrieved from *https://www.usp.org/compounding/general-chapter-hazardous-drugs-handling-healthcare*

What is patient-centered care?. (2017). *NEJM Catalyst.* Retrieved from https://catalyst.nejm.org/what-is-patient-centered-care/

3

Applying the DNP
Essentials to Practice

*"The growing number of DNP graduates presents a great poten-
tial for innovation around new care delivery models, interdisciplinary projects, and community involvement for a healthier
society."—Todd E. Tussing, DNP, RN, CENP, NEA-BC*

INTRODUCTION

The American Association of Colleges of Nursing (AACN) developed
a position statement in 2004 on the doctorate of nursing practice
(DNP; AACN, 2004). The concept of a doctorate in nursing that was
rooted in practice was not a new idea, as there had been other programs with different names since the late 1970s. However, the climate
of the healthcare industry was changing in the new millennium, and
nursing needed to respond in order to remain a thriving and growing
profession with input into the changes as they were occurring.

THE INSTITUTE OF MEDICINE REPORTS OF THE EARLY 2000s

The Institute of Medicine (IOM) has investigated and reported on
a multitude of problems and issues in the healthcare arena. We will

discuss those from the late 1990s and early 2000s that influenced the development and growth of the DNP degree in the United States. In 1999, the report on medical errors, *To Err Is Human: Building a Safer Health System* (Kohn, Corrigan, & Donaldson, 2000), was released to the public by the IOM. This report focused on the cost, both human and monetary, of medical errors and the factors contributing to these errors. In 2001, the IOM (Committee on Quality Health Care in America, 2001) released its report, *Crossing the Quality Chasm*, which focused on the inefficient use of resources, again both human and monetary, as well as physical resources in the healthcare system. This report also discussed the need for all care to be client/patient centered and safe. There were two reports released by the IOM in 2003, both of which addressed nursing issues. The first, *Health Professions Education: A Bridge to Quality*, spoke to the need for the education of nurses and other healthcare professionals to be focused on and pointed to educating professionals who would be able to deliver patient-centered care in a multidisciplinary model with a focus on evidence-based principles, quality indicators (QI), and technology (Greiner, & Knebel, 2003). The second report in 2003 was *Keeping Patients Safe and Transforming the Work Environment of Nurses* (Page, 2004). Changes in the healthcare industry had drastically changed the leadership landscape within institutions. This report focused on the need of healthcare organizations to have the best prepared clinical leaders at all levels of management to participate in executive decisions. Nursing needed to assure that there would be nursing leaders "at the table" as called for by that latest IOM report.

Fast Facts

One of nursing's response to these reports and the rapidly changing healthcare environment was the development of an AACN task force. This task force was tasked with among other items developing strategies to address the issues brought forward by the various IOM reports. One of the outcomes of this task force was the development of the position statement on the DNP, a terminal degree

(continued)

(continued)

in practice of nursing to complement the PhD in nursing, which was focused on generating new nursing knowledge. This statement was then utilized to make recommendations on the future of practice-focused doctorate education—both in the development of curricular requirements and the implementation of the role.

The Position Paper

The position paper delineated the context in which the practice-based doctorate would be defined and differentiated from the research doctorate in nursing as a second terminal degree with equal footing, the nomenclature to be utilized when describing the roles and responsibilities, and that it would prepare graduates for the highest level of nursing practice. Initially, the DNP degree was narrowly defined as being the entry to practice level for nurse practitioners. However, as time went on, other nurses in advanced roles in leadership and academics began to show interest in the new programs as they were developing. Nurses who were not nurse practitioners but were in an advanced nursing role saw the DNP degree as a valuable addition to their education that would add to their practice. This may not have been the initial intent of the DNP degree, as nurses inhabit many roles, all of which are components of the practice of nursing; therefore, the DNP degree has already expanded from its initial intent to include all of these aspects of nursing.

The DNP Curriculum

The position statement also set forth the areas of content for practice-based doctoral programs to utilize when educating those nurses who chose this path to a terminal degree. The areas of content are eight in number and follow the template of the other educational levels in nursing, and they became known as the Essentials of DNP Education (AACN, 2006). As programs are developed all over the United States, and abroad, the Essentials are used to frame the curriculum and develop courses.

The Essentials set forth by the AACN are as follows:

I. Scientific Underpinnings for Practice
II. Organizational and Systems Leadership for Quality Improvement and Systems Thinking
III. Clinical Scholarship and Analytical Methods for Evidence-Based Practice
IV. Information Systems/Technology and Patient Care Technology for the Improvement and Transformation of Health Care
V. Health Care Policy for Advocacy in Health Care
VI. Inter-Professional Collaboration for Improving Patient and Population Health Outcomes
VII. Clinical Prevention and Population Health for Improving the Nation's Health
VIII. Advanced Nursing Practice (AACN, 2006).

One of the most obvious ways to establish whether or not those with DNP degrees are actually employing the Essentials and demonstrating the competencies is to examine the literature written about the DNP degree. The types of research that are emphasized in practice-based doctoral programs are (a) evidence-based research as it directly relates to practice and (b) translational research of primary research to practice. Evidence-based practice was introduced by Dr. Rosenberg and Dr. Donald as a system of using evidence rather than "history" to make clinical decisions and thereby improve outcomes and the validity of science (Rosenberg & Donald, 1995). It was the prevailing thought of these two physicians that having evidence that an intervention was the right course of action was better than doing something to patients because "that's how we've always done it." This then began to seep into the other health professions as a viable way of providing care that would lead to better outcomes. In order to become an expert in evidence-based practice, DNP-prepared nurses need to become proficient and expert at evaluating and utilizing research.

DNP Competencies

These same Essentials inform and define the competencies that are at the core of all advanced nursing practice. Each Essential has competencies associated with it. The competencies define which behaviors each individual nurse should exhibit when employing that Essential in his or her individual practice. The competencies are such that all nurses in advanced roles will be able to employ the competencies in their daily practice, whether they are clinical practitioners, educators, leaders, administrators, or informatics specialists.

DNP-prepared nurses must possess skills that would allow them to both design and implement evidence-based projects. The skills required by the DNP-prepared nurses to accomplish this specific aspect of care provided to individuals and populations are a working knowledge of the process of evidence-based practice, the ability and expertise to search and utilize databases, and expertise in the ability to critically appraise current evidence and then apply the findings to varied situations to improve patient care outcomes (Rojjanasrirat & Rice, 2017).

Fast Facts

It is not enough to be able to espouse the Essentials as written by the AACN. Nurses who are educationally prepared with and earn a DNP must be able to apply the Essentials to their daily practice, synthesize evidence, apply evidence to initiate change, and communicate the best evidence—they must live them.

We will look at each of these competencies in relation to the Essentials with which they are associated and provide examples of how DNP-prepared nurses may exemplify them.

ESSENTIAL I: SCIENTIFIC UNDERPINNINGS FOR PRACTICE

This Essential states nursing is a practice discipline that is based on scientific principles. Nursing draws from the natural and social sciences as well as established and emerging nursing science. Much of the nursing science utilized by DNP-prepared nurses falls in the category of middle-range theory (AACN, 2006).

Competencies Associated With Essential I

The DNP graduate will be able to:

1. Integrate nursing science with knowledge from ethics and the biophysical, psychosocial, analytical, and organizational sciences as the basis for the highest level of nursing practice.

2. Use science-based theories and concepts to determine the nature and significance of health and healthcare delivery phenomena; describe the actions and advanced strategies to enhance, alleviate, and ameliorate health and healthcare delivery phenomena as appropriate; and evaluate outcomes.
3. Develop and evaluate new practice approaches based on nursing theories and theories from other disciplines.

The competencies of Essential I set the foundation for advanced nursing practice to be broad in its approach and perspective. This is accomplished by drawing from associated knowledge from various disciplines. The DNP-prepared nurses must be experts in the application and evaluation of nursing and nonnursing theories to provide the best outcomes for the patient, community, or population they are serving.

Examples of Roles Associated With Essential I Competencies

- An APRN using the Nightingale's environmental theory along with the family systems theory when providing care to a patient at home with multiple chronic health problems
- A nurse administrator utilizing the systems or organizational theory when evaluating organizational-wide staffing problems
- A nurse educator utilizing various learning theories in the classroom to ensure nursing content is being presented in a way that is in accordance with accepted educational practice

ESSENTIAL II: ORGANIZATIONAL AND SYSTEMS LEADERSHIP FOR QUALITY IMPROVEMENT AND SYSTEMS THINKING

This Essential addresses DNP-prepared nurses' abilities and appropriateness to occupy leadership roles and positions. These can range from informal leaders to formal C-suite roles (AACN, 2006).

Competencies Associated With Essential II

The DNP graduate will be able to:

1. Develop and evaluate care delivery approaches that meet current and future needs of patient populations based on scientific findings in nursing and other clinical sciences, as well as organizational, political, and economic sciences.

2. Ensure accountability for quality of healthcare and patient safety for populations with whom they work.

   a. Use advanced communication skills/processes to lead quality improvement and patient safety initiatives in healthcare systems
   b. Employ principles of business, finance, economics, and health policy to develop and implement effective plans for practice-level and/or system-wide practice initiatives that will improve the quality of care delivery
   c. Develop and/or monitor budgets for practice initiatives
   d. Analyze the cost-effectiveness of practice initiatives accounting for risk and improvement of healthcare outcomes
   e. Demonstrate sensitivity to diverse organizational cultures and populations, including patients and providers

3. Develop and/or evaluate effective strategies for managing the ethical dilemmas inherent in patient care, the healthcare organization, and research.

Examples of Roles Associated With Essential II

- A DNP–APRN notes that there is poor flow in the clinic in which she or he works. The APRN then takes on the responsibility of investigating the problem and finding a solution. This is informal leadership.
- A DNP-prepared nurse is hired to fill the position of joint chief nursing officer and chief clinical officer. This is formal leadership.
- A DNP-prepared educator is asked to chair a committee at the college where they work to evaluate a problem with the hiring of new faculty.
- A DNP-prepared nurse informaticist develops a streamlined system for charting with an electronic medical record.
- A DNP-prepared nurse is hired as the administrative head of a hospital department.

ESSENTIAL III: CLINICAL SCHOLARSHIP AND ANALYTICAL METHODS FOR EVIDENCE-BASED PRACTICE

This Essential speaks to the ability of a DNP-prepared nurse to evaluate, translate, integrate, and apply evidence-based practice for the purpose of improved outcomes. The practice focus of DNP-prepared nurses provides them with the ability to effectively connect practice with science, caring, and human needs and then evaluate the situation and outcomes (AACN, 2006).

Competencies Associated With Essential III

The DNP graduate will be able to:

1. Use analytic methods to critically appraise existing literature and other evidence to determine and implement the best evidence for practice.
2. Design and implement processes to evaluate outcomes of practice, practice patterns, and systems of care within a practice setting, healthcare organization, or community against national benchmarks to determine variances in practice outcomes and population trends.
3. Design, direct, and evaluate quality improvement methodologies to promote safe, timely, effective, efficient, equitable, and patient-centered care.
4. Apply relevant findings to develop practice guidelines and improve practice and the practice environment.
5. Use information technology and research methods appropriately to collect appropriate and accurate data to generate evidence for nursing practice; inform and guide the design of databases that generate meaningful evidence for nursing practice; analyze data from practice; design evidence-based interventions; predict and analyze outcomes; examine patterns of behavior and outcomes; and identify gaps in evidence for practice.
6. Function as a practice specialist/consultant in collaborative knowledge-generating research.
7. Disseminate findings from evidence-based practice and research to improve healthcare outcomes.

Examples of Roles Associated With Essential III

- A DNP-prepared nurse notes a chronic patient care problem and does a literature search to ascertain if this is a problem about which someone has written.

- A DNP-prepared nurse pairs with a nurse researcher to conduct a study on the identified patient care problem.
- A guideline is developed by the DNP-prepared nurse based on the results of study.

ESSENTIAL IV: INFORMATION SYSTEMS/TECHNOLOGY AND PATIENT CARE TECHNOLOGY FOR THE IMPROVEMENT AND TRANSFORMATION OF HEALTH CARE

This Essential addresses the DNP-prepared nurse's ability to use information technology to improve patient outcomes, assist in clinical decision-making, and support leadership goals of the institution (AACN, 2006).

Competencies Associated With Essential IV

The DNP graduate will be able to:

1. Design, select, use, and evaluate programs that evaluate and monitor outcomes of care, care systems, and quality improvement including consumer use of healthcare information systems.
2. Analyze and communicate critical elements necessary to the selection, use, and evaluation of healthcare information systems and patient care technology.
3. Demonstrate the conceptual ability and technical skills to develop and execute an evaluation plan involving data extraction from practice information systems and databases.
4. Provide leadership in the evaluation and resolution of ethical and legal issues within healthcare systems relating to the use of information, information technology, communication networks, and patient care technology.
5. Evaluate consumer health information sources for accuracy, timeliness, and appropriateness.

Examples of Roles Associated With Essential IV

- A DNP-prepared nurse works for a medical software company evaluating the nursing documentation sections of the software.

- A DNP-prepared nurse works for a government agency using data mining to identify trends in patient care.
- A DNP-prepared nurse works for a large hospital system reviewing trends identified through online communication with patients.

ESSENTIAL V: HEALTH CARE POLICY FOR ADVOCACY IN HEALTH CARE

Essential V speaks about the need for DNP-prepared nurses to be integrally involved with the development of and understand the connection between healthcare policy, advocacy, and practice (AACN, 2006). As practice-based professionals, this is a perfect fit for DNP graduates.

Competencies Associated With Essential V

The DNP graduate will be able to:

1. Critically analyze health policy proposals, health policies, and related issues from the perspective of consumers, nursing, other health professions, and other stakeholders in policy and public forums.
2. Demonstrate leadership in the development and implementation of institutional, local, state, federal, and/or international health policy.
3. Influence policy makers through active participation on committees, boards, or task forces at the institutional, local, state, regional, national, and/or international levels to improve healthcare delivery and outcomes.
4. Educate others, including policy makers at all levels, regarding nursing, health policy, and patient care outcomes.
5. Advocate for the nursing profession within the policy and healthcare communities.
6. Develop, evaluate, and provide leadership for healthcare policy that shapes healthcare financing, regulation, and delivery.
7. Advocate for social justice, equity, and ethical policies within all healthcare arenas.

Examples of Roles Associated With Essential V

- A DNP-prepared nurse serves on the board of a hospital.
- A DNP-prepared nurse works for a healthcare lobbying firm.
- A DNP-prepared nurse volunteers to be on a committee that analyzes public healthcare policies.
- A DNP nurse chairs a committee that is responsible for the visibility of nurses in the state.

ESSENTIAL VI: INTER-PROFESSIONAL COLLABORATION FOR IMPROVING PATIENT AND POPULATION HEALTH OUTCOMES

This Essential is an integral aspect of all levels of nursing as we are often the coordinators of care making it mandatory to interact and collaborate with other disciplines. The DNP-prepared nurse is viewed as an expert or leader in this area—bringing all necessary voices to the table (AACN, 2006).

Competencies Associated With Essential VI

The DNP graduate will be able to:

1. Employ effective communication and collaborative skills in the development and implementation of practice models, peer review, practice guidelines, health policy, standards of care, and/or other scholarly products.
2. Lead interprofessional teams in the analysis of complex practice and organizational issues.
3. Employ consultative and leadership skills with intraprofessional and interprofessional teams to create change in healthcare and complex healthcare delivery systems.

Examples of Roles Associated With Essential VI

- A DNP-prepared nurse is charged with developing and chairing a committee to evaluate a multidisciplinary patient care problem.
- A DNP-prepared nurse educator is hired to act as the head of a new department charged with educating medical students and nursing students together via simulation.

ESSENTIAL VII: CLINICAL PREVENTION AND POPULATION HEALTH FOR IMPROVING THE NATION'S HEALTH

Essential VII speaks to the ability of a DNP-prepared nurse to be intimately involved in population health issues, health promotion and prevention through the gathering of, and evaluation of, data in the spheres of environment, epidemiology, occupation, and biostatistics (AACN, 2006).

Competencies Associated With Essential VII

The DNP graduate will be able to:

1. Analyze epidemiological, biostatistical, environmental, and other appropriate scientific data related to individual, aggregate, and population health.
2. Synthesize concepts, including psychosocial dimensions and cultural diversity, related to clinical prevention and population health in developing, implementing, and evaluating interventions to address health promotion/disease prevention efforts, improve health status/access patterns, and/or address gaps in care of individuals, aggregates, or populations.
3. Evaluate care delivery models and/or strategies using concepts related to community, environmental and occupational health, and cultural and socioeconomic dimensions of health.

Examples of Roles Associated With Essential VII

- A DNP-prepared nurse is hired to evaluate community health needs as a hospital system prepares to expand clinics in the surrounding area.
- A DNP-prepared nurse is charged with evaluating the needs of the community in regard to health education to improve patient outcomes.

ESSENTIAL VIII: ADVANCED NURSING PRACTICE

This Essential speaks to the specialized clinical knowledge a DNP-prepared nurse has as it relates to a specific patient population.

DNP-prepared nurses are expected to develop therapeutic relationships with patients and other professionals with the goal of improved patient care, assessment, and outcomes (AACN, 2006).

Competencies Associated With Essential VIII

The DNP graduate will be able to:

1. Conduct a comprehensive and systematic assessment of health and illness parameters in complex situations, incorporating diverse and culturally sensitive approaches.
2. Design, implement, and evaluate therapeutic interventions based on nursing science and other sciences.
3. Develop and sustain therapeutic relationships and partnerships with patients (individual, family, or group) and other professionals to facilitate optimal care and patient outcomes.
4. Demonstrate advanced levels of clinical judgment, systems thinking, and accountability in designing, delivering, and evaluating evidence-based care to improve patient outcomes.
5. Guide, mentor, and support other nurses to achieve excellence in nursing practice.
6. Educate and guide individuals and groups through complex health and situational transitions.
7. Use conceptual and analytical skills in evaluating the links among practice, organizational, population, fiscal, and policy issues.

Examples of Roles Associated With Essential VIII

- A DNP-prepared nurse is hired to care for migrant farmers in a mobile clinic.
- A DNP-prepared nurse is hired by a school for special needs children to assist families in transitioning their children to the world as they approach the end of the program.
- A DNP-prepared nurse is hired by a private practice to develop a case-load of primary patients.
- A DNP-prepared nurse is hired by an urban urgicenter to see patients in the off-hours for emergencies.

SUMMARY

The competencies as described by the AACN Essentials of the DNP provide a framework for the type of work someone who completes a DNP program may choose to pursue. They are broad enough to allow for multiple opportunities both in and out of nursing as a base of operations.

Fast Facts

The unifying concept for all of the competencies is the patient and improving outcomes for that patient whether it is an individual, a family, a community, a population, or the population of the world. This is a brave new world for the practice doctorate. Welcome to it!

REFLECTION QUESTIONS

1. Do you feel the Essentials, as developed and implemented, encompass all aspects of advanced nursing practice or are there aspects that should not be included and others that are not delineated?

2. Which competencies do you feel are the most important for a DNP-prepared nurse in a clinical role to possess and to manifest skill?

3. Which competencies do you believe to be the most important for a DNP-prepared nurse to possess and to manifest skill when in the role of educator?

4. Which competencies do you believe to be the most important for a DNP-prepared nurse to possess and to manifest skill when in the role of an administrator?

5. Choose six competencies and reflect on how a DNP-prepared APRN, nurse educator, and nurse administrator would use each of them.

6. Which DNP competencies would you anticipate utilizing, and what would the outcomes of that utilization be, in a role you anticipate inhabiting after the completion of your DNP program?

References

American Association of Colleges of Nursing. (2004). *AACN position statement on the practice doctorate in nursing.* Retrieved from https://www.aacnnursing.org/Portals/42/News/Position-Statements/DNP.pdf

American Association of Colleges of Nursing. (2006). *The essentials of doctoral education for advanced nursing practice.* Retrieved from https://www.aacnnursing.org/Portals/42/Publications/DNPEssentials.pdf

Committee on Quality Health Care in America. (2001). *Crossing the quality chasm: A new health system for the 21st century.* Washington, DC: National Academies Press. Retrieved from https://www.ncbi.nlm.nih.gov/pubmed/25057539

Greiner, A., & Knebel, E. (Eds.). (2003). *Health professions education: A bridge to quality.* Washington, DC: National Academies Press. Retrieved from https://www.ncbi.nlm.nih.gov/books/NBK221528

Kohn, L. T., Corrigan, J. M., & Donaldson, M. S. (Eds.). (2000). *To Err is human: Building a safer health system.* Washington, DC: National Academies Press. Retrieved from https://www.ncbi.nlm.nih.gov/books/NBK225182

Page, A. (Ed.). (2004). *Keeping patients safe: Transforming the work environment of nurses.* Washington, DC: National Academies Press. Retrieved from https://www.ncbi.nlm.nih.gov/books/NBK216190

Rojjanasrirat, W., & Rice, J. (2017). Evidenced-based practice knowledge, attitudes and practice of online graduate students. *Nurse Education Today, 53,* 48–53. doi:10.1016/j.nedt.2017.04.005

Rosenberg, W., & Donald, A. (1995). Evidence-based medicine: An approach to clinical problem-solving. *British Medical Journal, 310,* 1122–1126. doi:10.1136/bmj.310.6987.1122

II

Roles for the DNP

4

Juxtaposition of the DNP

"The journey of completing the DNP degree has allowed me to see the nursing profession from a broader perspective. I learned how we can impact our practice through affective change, as well as how to best coach and mentor staff through the complex change."—Kimberly Rivera, DNP, RN-BC, OCN

INTRODUCTION

The Art of Practicing

Addressing the foundation of nursing is paramount before delving into the doctor of nursing practice (DNP) degree. The fundamentals of nursing are to provide high-quality care to anyone who has fallen acutely or chronically ill. The World Health Organization elegantly describes *nursing* as encompassing "autonomous and collaborative care of individuals of all ages, families, groups and communities, sick or well and in all settings. It includes the promotion of health, the prevention of illness, and the care of ill, disabled and dying people" (n.d., para. 1) This is a simple but accurate definition and highlights the key aspects of nursing care.

Most of us are taught at an early age from parents and family members that if one takes time practicing, one can become proficient and/or master a specific subject, project, or sport. The concept of practicing can be related to any academic subject, such as math,

English, and science, as well as athletics and arts. Specific examples include calculus, algebra, soccer, basketball, dance, and playing a musical instrument. More importantly, nursing is not exempted from this elementary concept of practicing. Nursing professors preach at great lengths to nursing students: "Please practice your nursing skills. Please practice your NCLEX® questions." The skills range from basic bed-making to advanced health assessment. The foundation of most nursing programs includes:

1. Nursing fundamental procedures
   a. Foley catheters
   b. Trach care and suctioning
   c. Medication administration
   d. Wound care and sterile gloving
2. Health assessment
   a. Head-to-toe bedside assessment
   b. Advanced health assessment
3. National Council Licensure Exam (NCLEX) questions (the dreaded questions, but a necessary evil!)

Fast Facts

These procedures and test-taking techniques have been drilled and practiced at great lengths. Those who master these skills tend to be nurses who provide consistent high-quality care. Nurses never move away from practicing their skills, expertise, and knowledge no matter how long in the profession. Therefore, the process of continuing to practice skills and enhance knowledge can be transferred to multiple role options for the DNP.

NURSING PRACTICE

Nursing practice is the pinnacle theory for the DNP. The terms *nursing* and *practice* are two key words that blend together and morph into the framework of nursing. Nursing practice can be described by the way in which every single nurse delivers high-quality, safe care to patients, regardless of the role or title.

The nurse practice act governs the way nurses deliver care and may vary from state to state. The nurse practice act has specific legal statutes that are determined by each state legislature. The act is responsible for determining the scope of practice for each nurse within the designated state.

Nurses must be astutely aware of their state's practice act and remember that the practice act was created to protect the public from harm. The American Nurses Association elegantly describes the scope of nursing practice as the "who," "what," "where," "when," "why," and "how."

The Ws of the scope of practice can be interpreted as the following:

- "Who" means the accurate title of the professional nurse. The nurse must hold an active and current license.
- "What" is related to the fundamentals of nursing. It involves all the aspects of delivering safe, high-quality care.
- "Where" means the ability to deliver care in any situation in which an individual is deemed or identified as a patient.
- "When" refers to the need of a nurse's knowledge, expertise, skill, and kindness.
- "Why" refers to the goals of delivering high-quality care and patient outcomes.

This description of the nursing scope of practice can be applied to each nurse regardless of the role within the nursing profession.

UNDERSTANDING JUXTAPOSITION

Now that the basic concepts of nursing and nursing practice have been reviewed, many may be thinking: What is meant by the juxtaposition of the DNP? *Juxtaposition* can be explained as the ability to compare and contrast two items, subjects, and/or situations.

The juxtaposition of the DNP role is related to the fact that DNP education is identified as a terminal degree that focuses on nursing practice. The concept of nursing practice in this case has been interrupted in various ways since the inception of the degree, hence causing the juxtaposition.

The DNP degree was initially created for the advanced practice roles in nursing. The American Association of Colleges of Nursing task force developed the DNP degree to be the terminal doctoral degree for advanced practice registered nurses (APRNs), which emphasized nurse practitioners (NPs). The doctoral degree set precedence for other disciplines, such as physical and occupational therapy, to elevate advanced practice healthcare providers with a terminal practice degree.

To date, there has been an unexpected major shift in nurses who are applying for and obtaining the practice doctoral degree. The momentum in which the DNP degree has attracted nurses from all roles, specialties, and settings has significantly changed the environment in which it was initially derived. Table 4.1 demonstrates the comparison and contrast of the intended and current use of the DNP.

Table 4.1

Juxtaposition of the DNP: Intended Use Versus Current Use of DNP Programs

Intended DNP Programs	Current DNP Programs
DNP education for APRNs—NPs	DNP education for all nurses who want to pursue a doctoral degree
Marketed to NPs	Marketed to all nurses
Focus on the DNP Essentials	Focus on the DNP Essentials
Traditional advanced practice roles Direct patient care	Nontraditional nursing roles Indirect patient care
Major focus on advanced practice competencies	Diverse focus on multiple competencies (depending on individual nursing role and university programs)
Advanced practice role for the DNP project with diversity in the specialty nursing area	Diverse focus on the project depends on the specialty area of DNP students
Some DNP programs accept only APRNs/NPs	Some DNP programs accept non-APRNs/NPs
Enhance nursing practice/leadership skills	Enhance nursing practice/leadership skills

(continued)

Table 4.1

Juxtaposition of the DNP: Intended Use Versus Current Use of DNP Programs (*continued*)	
Intended DNP Programs	**Current DNP Programs**
APRN/NP educators only	Non-NP educators
End point goal for a terminal degree	End point goal for a terminal degree
	Continuing to evolve
Advanced practice nursing career pathways	Potential for numerous nursing career pathways
	– Administration
	– Education
	– Entrepreneurial

NP, nurse practitioner.

CHANGE IN VISION OF THE DNP

The vision of the DNP student is no longer isolated to APRNs, such as NPs. The magnetism to the practice aspect has enticed not just APRN/NPs but nurses from other disciplines, such as education and administration. It is evident by the increasing number of both DNP programs and nurses who have completed the degree requirements. It is imperative to recognize that not every DNP will be an APRN/NP. Nurses from all specialties are pursuing the DNP, such as the following:

1. Medical/surgical nurses
2. Oncology nurses
3. Critical care nurses
4. Labor and delivery nurses
5. ED nurses
6. Operative nurses
7. Adult NPs
    a. Adult geriatrics
    b. Family
    c. Pediatrics
8. Chief nursing officers
9. Nursing managers and directors

10. Educators
    a. Academic educators
    b. Staff development/nurse educators

The preceding list is just a sample of the types of nurses who are pursuing the DNP degree, to illustrate its appeal to a wide cross-section of nurses.

BENEFITS OF DNP NURSES

Nurses, administrators, and healthcare system leaders need to acknowledge the skill set of DNP graduates. Organizations need to encourage, create, and allow DNP-prepared nurses to function in traditional and nontraditional nursing roles. Tussing et al. (2018) identified and supported the view that "the growing number of DNP graduates presents a great potential for innovation around new care delivery models, interdisciplinary projects, and community involvement for a healthier society" (p. 602). Therefore, the wealth of knowledge, leadership skills, systems theory and concepts, and advanced practice abilities can positively and significantly add to and/or change healthcare delivery methods.

Fast Facts

Leaders and organizations need to be cognizant of the value of the DNP and be open to new and redesigned roles.

As the DNP-prepared nurse evolves, the following will be valued and recognized:

1. Healthcare systems and organization will have increased numbers of DNP graduates who function as administrators and healthcare leaders.
2. There will be an increased opportunity to have a better understanding of the advantages for DNP-prepared nurses within a healthcare organization.
3. DNP-prepared nurses will have multiple career choices from which to choose within a healthcare system and be utilized appropriately.

4. There is potential for patients and family members to have increased knowledge of the advantages of DNP-prepared nurses.
5. There will be creation of innovative roles for DNP nurses.

DNP SKILLS MATCH DNP ESSENTIALS

Another important factor to understand is that the skills acquired by DNP-prepared nurses coincide with the DNP Essentials. The Essentials are the foundation of the DNP degree. The DNP students can choose from the wide array of competencies that can be tailored to their project, new role, and/or new title. Using the DNP Essentials and new skill sets will assist the DNP-prepared nurse to perform within the changing healthcare environment and deliver high-quality care to a diverse patient population, as well as engage in leadership, organizational, and system concepts.

DNP programs have embraced the diversity of the DNP student by creating cohorts of NPs, administrators, and educators. DNP programs promote the DNP Essentials and acknowledge the skills and qualities a DNP-prepared nurse needs to cultivate and master in order to be successful and navigate within the current healthcare system. Here is an outline of the skills and qualities necessary for DNP-prepared nurses:

1. Understanding and implementing leadership skills at multiple levels
   a. Leadership qualities
   b. Mentorship qualities
   c. Advanced critical thinking
2. Understanding an overview of global health issues
   a. Infectious diseases concerns
   b. Vaccine controversies
   c. Underserved and compromised patient populations
3. Understanding the impact of financial issues
   a. Cost of medications and procedures
   b. Patient insurance coverage concerns
   c. Resources available for healthcare personnel
4. Understanding the importance of advanced nursing assessments
   a. Advanced health assessment skills
   b. Performing advanced procedures

    c. Critical thinking skills

    d. Being an expert in specialty area

    e. Certifications

5. Awareness of healthcare policy

    a. Legal aspects

    b. Ethical aspects

    c. Current political issues

        i. New policies and laws

        ii. Current with appropriate state nursing practice act

6. Recognition of educational variations for DNP nurses

    a. Academia roles

        i. Tenured track

        ii. Nontenured track

    b. Staff development role

        i. Acute care setting

        ii. Long-term care setting

    c. Consultant roles

7. Understanding the importance of patient care outcomes

    a. Decrease of readmission rates

    b. Decrease in hospital-acquired infections

    c. Increase in patient satisfaction scores

    d. National benchmarks

    e. Patient safety goals

8. Understanding of organizations and healthcare system issues

    a. Costs of healthcare

        i. Patients

        ii. Staff

        iii. Systems

    b. Available resources

    c. Reimbursement concerns

        i. Governmental implications

        ii. Private insurance implications

    d. Global insurance collaborations

9. Understanding current standards and area for change with nursing practice setting

    a. Identification and implementation

        i. Quality and performance improvement projects

        ii. Evidence-based practice projects

        iii. Research projects

10. Recognizing informatics challenges
    a. Use of appropriate computerized order entry
    b. Safety of computerized ordering
    c. Identification of medication errors
        i. Rectifying medication issues
        ii. Preventing medication errors

Fast Facts

Nurses have realized the benefits and advantages that the DNP degree can offer. More importantly, nurses need to understand and perfect the qualities and skills needed as a DNP-prepared nurse.

WHERE THE DNP NURSE FITS INTO THE HEALTHCARE SYSTEM

Some might be questioning, Where does a DNP-prepared nurse fit? How do DNP nurses make the public aware of the role? How does a DNP eliminate potential role confusion? What can you do with the DNP degree? The questions can be endless, but so can the answers. Although these are thought-provoking questions, the solutions are easy with three simple steps.

1. Explain the advantages of the DNP preparation.
    a. Patients
    b. Families
    c. Leaders
    d. Healthcare colleagues
2. Practice clear communication.
    a. Clarify misconceptions
    b. Answer questions
3. Market DNP appropriately.
    a. Prepare consistent introduction
    b. Demonstrate excellent assessment skills
    c. Manifest professionalism
    d. Display confidence

The nurse with a DNP degree can apply for jobs in various areas of healthcare and patient care in a multitude of roles. Obtaining the DNP degree can open pathways to fascinating, interesting, traditional, and nontraditional nursing positions. The next phase is to

Table 4.2

Professional Role Options for the DNP-Prepared Nurse: Direct Patient Care

Potential DNP Nursing Roles	Professional Pathways	DNP Skill Sets (Based on the DNP Essentials)
Direct patient care nurse—staff nurse*	– Private offices	**Essential I**
Specialty areas	– Large and small healthcare systems	– Excellent assessment skills
– Primary care	– Insurance companies	**Essential II**
– Critical care	– Long-term care organizations	– Leadership skills
– Oncology		– Mentorship skills
– Rehabilitation	– Elementary and high school districts	**Essential III**
– Palliative care		– Evidence-based practice skills
– Medical/surgical		**Essential IV**
– Transplant		– Informatics skills
– Bone marrow/ stem cell		– Order entry
– Renal		– MAR documentation
– Pediatrics		**Essential V**
– Geriatrics		– Understanding current health policy
– Women's health		**Essential VII**
		– Financial impact to patients and organization
		– Available resources
		– Current health problems
		Essential VIII
		– Advanced practice skills

*There are some DNP nurses who continue to function as staff nurses. (This role should be welcomed as they are highly educated nurses at the forefront acting as informal leaders and mentors for colleagues and advocates for patients.)
MAR, medication administration record.

identify the career options that may be available for a DNP-prepared nurse. Tables 4.2 to 4.6 depict the potential opportunities for DNP-prepared nurses.

Table 4.3

Professional Role Options for the DNP-Prepared Nurse: Nurse Practitioners

Potential DNP Nursing Roles	Professional Pathways	DNP Skill Sets (Based on the DNP Essentials)

– Adult primary care
– Family
– Geriatrics
– Pediatrics
– Transplant
  – Bone marrow/
    stem cell
  – Renal
– Women's health
– Critical care
– Emergency
– Trauma
– Rehabilitation
– Palliative care
	– Private offices
	– Large and small
	  healthcare
	  organizations
	– Long-term care
	  organizations
	– Insurance companies
		Essential I
		  – Excellent assessment skills
		Essential II
		  – Leadership skills
		  – Mentorship skills
		Essential III
		  – Evidence-based practice skills
		  – Development of nursing research projects
		Essential IV
		  – Informatics skills
		    – Order entry
		    – MAR documentation
		Essential V
		  – Understanding current health policy
		Essential VI
		  – Manage working with multiple divisions and staff
		Essential VII
		  – Financial impact to patients and organization
		  – Available resources
		  – Current health problems
		Essential VIII
		  – Advanced practice skills

MAR, medication administration record.

Table 4.4

Professional Role Options for the DNP-Prepared Nurse: Education

Potential DNP Nursing Roles	Professional Pathways	DNP skill sets (Based on the DNP Essentials)
– Academia – Staff development	– Colleges and universities – Large and small healthcare organizations – Pharmaceutical/medical companies – Private healthcare organizations	**Essential I** – Excellent assessment skills **Essential II** – Leadership skills – Mentorship skills **Essential III** – Evidence-based practice skills – Development of nursing research projects – Educational advancement skills **Essential IV** – Informatics skills – Order entry – MAR documentation **Essential V** – Understanding current health policy **Essential VI** – Manage working with multiple divisions and staff **Essential VII** – Financial impact to patients and organization – Available resources – Current health problems **Essential VIII** – Advanced practice skills

MAR, medication administration record.

Table 4.5

Professional Role Options for the DNP-Prepared Nurse: Administration/Leadership Roles		
Potential DNP Nursing Roles	**Professional Pathways**	**DNP Skill Sets (Based on the DNP Essentials)**

– Chief nursing officers
– Director
– Nurse managers
– Magnet coordinators
	– Large and small healthcare organizations
	– Leaders in healthcare systems
		Essential II
		  – Leadership skills
		  – Motivational skills
		  – Mentorship skills
		  – System theories
		  – Financial resources
		    – Budgets
		    – Operations
		    – Staffing
		  – Group dynamic skills
		Essential III
		  – Evidence-based practice skills
		Essential V
		  – Understanding current health policy
		Essential VI
		  – Manage working with multiple divisions and staff
		Essential VII
		  – Financial impact to patients and organization
		  – Available resources
		  – Current health problems

Table 4.6

Professional Role Options for the DNP-Prepared Nurse: Entrepreneurial Roles

Potential DNP Nursing Roles	Professional Pathways	DNP Skill Sets (Based on the DNP Essentials)

– Independent consultants
– Authors
– Health industry
– ANCC positions
– Joint commission
– Magnet positions
– Pharmaceutical industry
– Legal and ethical roles
	– Healthcare systems
	– Authors/editors
	– Directors
	– Coordinators
	– Independent contractors
		Essential I
		  – Excellent assessment skills
		Essential II
		  – Leadership skills
		  – Mentorship skills
		  – Marketing skills
		Essential III
		  – Evidence-based practice skills
		  – Development of nursing research projects
		Essential IV
		  – Informatics skills
		  – Billing concepts
		Essential V
		  – Understanding current health policy
		  – Risk populations
		Essential VI
		  – Manage working with multiple divisions and staff
		  – Analysis of different organizations
		Essential VII
		  – Financial impact to patients and organization
		  – Available resources
		  – Current health problems
		  – Patient advocates skills

ANCC, American Nurses Credentialing Center.

LEADERSHIP

Although the degree was dedicated to the APRNs/NPs, the juxtaposition that the DNP degree can be incorporated into several nursing roles has created a unique environment for all to pursue the terminal degree. The increase in programs and a wide array of nursing opportunities have promoted the positive characteristics of the DNP-prepared nurses.

This chapter has provided an overview of nursing, nursing practice, and the trends in the development of the DNP degree. However, it would be remiss if the topic of leadership is not addressed. Newland (2017) commented "desired outcomes for DNP graduates include clinical leadership and clinical scholarship. Not all DNP graduates are engaged in direct patient care; some impact patient outcomes indirectly" (p. 5).

Leadership is essential for pursing the DNP degree and is a common theme within the literature and the DNP Essentials. The literature supports the roles and qualities of DNP nurses. Malloch (2017) stated "we need to push the walls of leadership to embrace the future in which incredible opportunities are regularly unveiled by higher level thinking" (p. 29). This author has clearly captured the DNP nurse. Leadership can be defined through many lenses. Leaders can learn, practice, and perform the following:

1. Inspire
2. Encourage
3. Support
4. Listen
5. Recognize strengths and weakness of colleagues
6. Communicate clearly
7. Control emotions
8. Establish objectives, goals, and expectations
9. Build trust
10. Strive to be fair
11. Think critically

Leadership Opportunities for DNP Nurses

1. Administration roles
   a. Unit managers
   b. Division directors
   c. System directors
   d. Magnet directors
      i. Charge of Magnet teams

2. Charge of team assignments/special projects
3. Pharmaceutical/medical projects
4. Educational leader
   a. Staff development
      i. Grand rounds
      ii. Writing grants/publications
      iii. Evidence-based projects/research
5. Entrepreneur
   a. Educational consultant
   b. Private tutoring
   c. Systems consultant
   d. Informatics leader

SUMMARY

This chapter provided an overview of the importance and understanding of nursing practice and how it applies to the DNP role. The DNP role was initially created for the APRN/NP, but over the past decade, nurses from different specialties have identified the personal and professional positive career options available. In summary, the chapter demonstrated the following:

1. The nurse practice act guides practice for all nurses—regardless of the nursing role.
2. There is a shift in DNP nurses pursuing a DNP degree.
3. Development and mastery of critical thinking skills are important.
4. DNP Essentials are the foundation of the DNP degree.
5. DNP-prepared nurses have numerous career opportunities.
6. Leadership qualities for DNP nurses are important.

REFLECTION QUESTIONS

1. How do you think the changes in the vision of the DNP-prepared nurse has/will change the delivery of healthcare?
2. What nursing role will best fit your professional goals as a DNP-prepared nurse?

(continued)

3. If you were an administrator, how would you plan to best utilize your DNP-prepared nurses within the organization?
4. What Essential skill set do you believe to be the most important for the roles you intend to explore?
5. How do you plan to address yourself with patients and other staff members? How do you believe your title will be perceived within your current organization?
6. What leadership qualities do you possess? What skills do you need to master?

References

Malloch, K. (2017). Leading DNP professionals practice competencies for organizational excellence and advancement. *Nursing Administration Quarterly, 41*, 29–38. doi:10.1097/NAQ.0000000000000200

Newland, J. (2017). The DNP in 2017. *The Nurse Practitioner, 16*, 4–5. doi:10.1097/01. NPR0000513342.59265.6e

Tussing, T., Brinkman, B., Francis, D., Hixon, B., Labardee, R., & Chipps, E. (2018). The impact of the doctor of nursing practice nurse in a hospital setting. *The Journal of Nursing Administration, 48*, 600–602. doi:10.1097/NNA.0000000000000688

World Health Organization. (n.d.). *Nursing*. Retrieved from https://www.who.int/topics/nursing/en/

Further Reading

American Association of Colleges of Nursing. (2006). *The essentials of doctoral education for advanced nursing practice*. Retrieved from https://www.aacnnursing.org/Portals/42/Publications/DNPEssentials.pdf

American Nursing Association. (n.d.). *Scope of practice*. Retrieved from https://www.nursingworld.org/practice-policy/scope-of-practice

Pritham, U., & White, P. (2017). Assessing DNP impact using program evaluations to capture healthcare system change. *The Nurse Practitioner, 41*, 44–53. doi:10.1097/01.NPR.0000481509.24736.c8

Smith, D. (2006). Is the burden worth the benefit of the doctorate of nursing (DNP) for NPs? *Nephrology Nursing Journal, 33*, 685–686.

5

The DNP-Prepared
Nurse as a Clinician

"I became a DNP nurse clinician because obtaining the DNP allowed the opportunity to hold one of the highest degrees in nursing and care for patients at the front line. Applying the DNP Essentials *to daily practice is empowering."*—Toni Tortorella Genova, DNP, APN-BC, RN, FNP-BC, NP-C

INTRODUCTION

The role of clinician, or direct care provider, for a doctor of nursing practice (DNP)-prepared nurse is the least controversial of the roles currently embodied by nurses who hold the degree of DNP. The reason for this is simple: Advanced practice registered nurses (APRNs) were the intended population for the attainment of the degree since its inception. In 2004, the American Association of Colleges of Nursing (AACN) recommended the DNP as the practice-focused terminal degree in nursing for APRNs (AACN, 2004). Some noted healthcare trends that helped inform this decision are the increasing complexity of the U.S. healthcare system, large numbers of the aging baby boomer generation, increasing numbers of the oldest-old (80+), more complex diagnostic modalities and treatments, and medical doctors moving toward more specialization away from general practice.

Fast Facts

APRNs are positioned to play a vital role in the changing health-care system of the United States and by extension in the health of this nation. Therefore, APRNs will need a more extensive, in-depth knowledge base to meet these future challenges in patient care, healthcare systems, education, technology, and population health. The DNP provides all of this while additionally placing the nurse at the same educational level as others on the interprofessional team and thereby balancing the power structure of the team.

ROLES AND SETTINGS

The direct care role is the one most familiar to APRNs, and increasingly to the public. Currently, the most recognized advanced practice role is that of a nurse practitioner (NP). However, the APRN Consensus Model recognizes four specific APRN roles in nursing (APRN Consensus Work Group and the National Council of State Boards of Nursing APRN Advisory Group, 2008):

- NP (with specialties such as adult-gerontology, primary care; adult-gerontology, acute care; family, women's health, and gender-related care; pediatrics, primary care; pediatrics, acute care; and others)
- Clinical nurse specialist (CNS)
- Certified nurse midwife (CNM)
- Certified registered nurse anesthetist (CRNA)

Nurses who chose these roles as their areas of practice were the focus of the position statement by the AACN, regarding the goal of a terminal practice-focused degree as the entry level of practice for all APRNs (AACN, 2004). It was originally suggested to be put in place by 2015. Though it has not occurred according to the original timetable, the DNP degree has become the most sought-after terminal degree for nurses. All nurses in the previously mentioned roles provide direct care to specific populations at a more advanced level.

It is important to also understand that nurses in these roles inhabit and function in other roles, such as in administration and education.

The vision was that in the rapidly changing healthcare system, APRNs would be an integral part of that change and work toward the maintenance or improvement of patient outcomes. It was anticipated that doctoral-prepared APRNs would continue to provide equivalent or improved care as did their master's-prepared counterparts, as evidenced by outcome analyses in more than one study (Kurtzman & Barnow, 2017; Laurant et al., 2018; Stanik-Hutt et al., 2013). In addition to the already-honed clinical skills and high-quality care, which are the hallmarks of APRN practice, doctoral level education, in the form of the DNP degree, provides for a direct care provider who can also deliver improved efficiency both at the patient and system level, share quality improvement initiatives, and identify emerging trends via evidence-based practice (EBP) translational research.

Looking at the added value of the doctoral-prepared APRN, one can envision an expanded direct caregiver role in multiple settings. Following are some examples, but clearly not all the possibilities, of the settings in which a DNP-prepared nurse can work and some of the roles in which they would function.

Acute Care Institutions

- Hospitalist
- NP (specialty NP on an interprofessional team, oncology, women's health and gender-related care, palliative care, psychiatric mental health, neonatal, pediatrics)
- Wound and ostomy care nurse (WOCN)
- CNS
- CNM
- CRNA

Medical Homes or Community Healthcare Center or Ambulatory Clinics

- Adult-gerontology, primary care
- Pediatric, primary care
- Family NP
- Psych NP
- CNM

- Women's health and gender-related care
- NP dermatology
- WOCN

Private Practices (Often Population Based)

- NP—multispecialty practice
- NP—single specialty
- CNM
- Pediatrics
- Psychiatric/mental health

Long-Term Care Facilities

- Adult-gerontology
- FNP
- WOCN

Entrepreneurship

The possibilities are endless and only limited by your imagination—and in some states collaborative practice agreements! So *please* know your state laws before embarking on a journey!

EDUCATIONAL CONSIDERATION

According to the DNP fact sheet of the AACN (AACN, 2019), there are 348 DNP program students in the United States, with 98 more in the planning stages as of March 2019. Of the 98 programs in the planning stage, 50 are postbaccalaureates and 48 are postmaster's in their design (AACN, 2019). DNP programs are offered in all 50 states and the District of Columbia. They are found in various formats:

Face-to-face instruction
Hybrid (a combination of face-to-face and online components)
Fully online instruction

All programs require a total of 1,000 clinical hours in both clinical and soft skills like leadership and policy. How those hours are accumulated and what activities "count" for clinical are school/

program dependent and should be a factor to be examined by prospective students when evaluating programs for application. The number of students both enrolled and graduated has also shown significant growth since the inception of the first program in 2006.

Fast Facts

In 2018, there were 32,678 enrolled DNP students and 7,039 DNP graduates in the United States compared with 29,093 and 6,090 in 2017 (AACN, 2019). Criticism of the DNP degree by some is that it will take students away from PhD programs. This, however, is not borne out by the numbers. The number of PhD programs has also increased but not nearly at the same pace as the DNP programs, and the number of enrolled students has remained relatively stable at approximately 700 to 800 (Campaign for Action, 2019).

The preceding statistics clearly indicate that the DNP degree and its focus on practice rather than research that leads to the development of new nursing knowledge, as is the focus of the PhD, have resonated with nurses across the country. Nursing has progressed, similar to other professions such as medicine, dentistry, pharmacy, psychology, physical therapy, and audiology, which require doctoral-level education for entry into practice.

DNP–APRN Recommendations, Not Mandates

As previously stated, the AACN adopted the position statement on the recommendation of doctoral-level educational preparation for APRNs to assist in the transformation of the healthcare system and improved outcomes for patients, which were called for by the Institute of Medicine (U.S.) Committee on the Health Professions Education Summit; Greiner, and Knebel (2003; AACN, 2004). With the DNP degree designed to focus on the application of knowledge to clinical practice, it is in this manner that patient outcomes will be positively impacted. However, the call for doctoral education for APRNs remains a recommendation and not a mandate for most categories of APRNs, which explain, to some extent, the two entry points for practice—the postbaccalaureate and postmaster's. A postmaster's option needs to remain available to allow all current APRNs who wish to pursue the DNP to do so, yet these programs continue to admit postbaccalaureate nurses who have no intention of obtaining a DNP. Pursuing a doctoral degree until it is mandated for all APRNs will depend on several factors, which include the following:

- A personal desire for advanced education
- A belief that this level of education has added value to patients
- Finances
- Career options
- Geographic location
- Availability of DNP faculty and preceptors

Some nurses may choose master's-level education as their sole APRN preparation. This does not mean they will not be fabulous APRNs in their respective specialties and roles. It may mean that in the future, they may not have as much mobility or choice in job opportunities. However, the nursing profession and DNP role are not at that point yet.

Fast Facts

Currently, master's-prepared and doctoral-prepared APRNs occupy similar spaces in the healthcare system. As time moves on, we may see changes in opportunities, making it more desirable for APRNs to obtain a DNP degree.

BSN to DNP

For those nurses who do not yet have master's-level education and are more forward-thinking, the postbaccalaureate DNP (BSN to DNP) may be a good choice. This type of program incorporates both the master's and DNP essentials and competencies into one program. It is more streamlined, avoiding some of the difficulties encountered when taking and completing two separate degrees—master's and then DNP. These nurses who are pursuing the highest clinical nursing degree will be prepared to meet or exceed current and future healthcare needs of patients, populations, systems, and policy-making. They will be the innovators of nursing's future. These nurses will be able to fill the gap in roles in nursing leadership, advanced clinical practice, administration, and faculty, which are all predicted by the U.S. Bureau of Labor Statistics(2019).

Some of the specializations offered by BSN to DNP programs are the following:

Direct patient care roles—APRNs

- Certified NP
- CNS
- CNM
- CRNA
- (CNS and NP also require the student to choose a population focus):
  1. Family/individual across the lifespan
  2. Adult-gerontology, primary or acute care
  3. Women's health/gender related
  4. Neonatal
  5. Pediatrics, primary or acute care
  6. Psychiatric/mental health

Systems/organizational/aggregate

- Administration
- Healthcare policy
- Informatics
- Information systems (Doctor of Nursing Practice DNP, n.d.)

NONSTANDARDIZED CERTIFICATION FOR DNP-PREPARED NURSES

Certification for APRNs, both master's prepared and DNP prepared, is not standardized at this point. There is some discussion as to whether there should be one exam that certifies basic knowledge and competencies of DNP-prepared nurses (Stanik-Hutt, 2008). It has been argued, however, that having a DNP exam would become another area in which there are multitiered nurses with the same degree and that there is not one valid exam that tests the competencies of the DNP-prepared nurse (Stanik-Hutt, 2008). Some APRNs are certified through the American Nurses Credentialing Center (ANCC), the American Association of NPs, and multiple specialty organizations, and some are not mandated to be certified.

CNSs are not certified through one organization or accrediting body. The National Association of Clinical Nurse Specialists (NACNS) approved a set of core competencies in 2010 for clinical specialists regardless of population served. These competencies are currently under revision to be available in 2019. In addition to the core competencies, there are specialized competencies delineated by specialty populations and academic degree attainment. These specialized areas are (NACNS, n.d.) the following:

- Adult-gerontology competencies
- Women's health competencies
- Core practice doctorate competencies

There are also a multitude of organizations including AACN and ANA that have endorsed these competencies (NACNS, 2011). CNSs can also be certified through specialty nurse organizations. One such organization is the Oncology Nursing Society that has an exam leading to a nurse who holds the title and credentials as an Oncology-Certified CNS.

The DNP-prepared certified NP is not educated to add to or increase the individual NP's clinical skill level. The National Organization of Nurse Practitioner Faculties (NONPF) has delineated an outline of skills expected from DNP-prepared NPs based on the Essentials of DNP education (Doctor of Nursing Practice DNP, n.d.). Areas of expertise associated with DNP-prepared NPs include the following:

- Scientific foundations of APRN leadership
- Quality of clinical practice inquiry
- Technology and information literacy
- Policy
- Healthcare delivery systems
- Ethics
- Independent practice

Fast Facts

The DNP-prepared NPs will possess increased organization, economic, and leadership skills, which will translate into change by bringing a systems perspective to clinical practice and increasingly complex treatment plans

Though there is currently no DNP certification, there are five different boards in the United States that award certification to nurses based on specific populations or practice focus (DeCapua, n.d.). The boards and their certifications are as follows:

- ANCC
  Adult-Gerontology, Acute Care   AGACNP-BC
  Adult-Gerontology, Primary Care   AGPCNP-BC
  Family   FNP-BC
  Psychiatric-Mental Health   PMHNP-BC
- Pediatric Nursing Certification Board (PNCB)
  Pediatric, Primary Care   CPNP-PC
  Pediatric, Acute Care   CPNP-AC
- National Certification Corporation (NCC)
  Neonatal   NNP-BC
  Women's Health Gender Related   WHNP-BC
- American Academy of Nurse Practitioners
  Certification Program (AANPCP)
  Family   FNP-C
  Adult-Gerontology, Primary Care   NP-C or ANP-
  Emergency   ENP-C
- American Association of Critical Care
  Nurses (AACCN)
  Adult-Gerontology, Acute Care   ACNPC-AG

CRNAs are the only group of nurses that will require the terminal clinical DNP degree as entry into practice. The date set at this time is by 2025, the DNP will be the entry to practice level of education (RegisteredNurseRN.com, n.d.). It was stated that the DNP degree would provide CRNAs with increased credibility and recognition of the high level of responsibility and knowledge necessary to administer anesthesia. CRNAs are certified through an exam administered by the NBCRNA. The credential used by certified registered nurse anesthetists is CRNA. As with other certified nurses, CRNAs can also specialize though there are no specialized exams or credentials based on populations or care areas.

CNMs have added areas of skill and knowledge to competency areas for those midwives with DNP degrees. Some of these new areas are the following:

- Leadership
- Educational and change theory
- Health policy
- Economics
- Midwifery

These skills and knowledge can only add to the practice of a midwife. Midwives had a history that was based on service to underserved populations, high-quality care to women and families, and innovative models of patient care and advocacy. At this time, there is no movement toward requiring a DNP degree for entry into or continued practice. Certification for nurse-midwives is administered by the American Midwifery Certification Board (n.d.). The credentials assigned after successful examination is CNM.

OPPORTUNITIES AND CHALLENGES

The challenge of the IOM report, *Health Professions Education: A Bridge to Quality* (Greiner & Knebel, 2003), was to build educational pathways for healthcare professionals, including nurses, that focused on providing safe, high-quality care. Some strategies outlined in the report were evidence-based care, teamwork among professionals, patient-centered care, information technology, and quality control. One way in which nursing answered this challenge was to put forward the recommendation that APRNs entering the workforce have an earned practice-focused doctorate (AACN, 2004). This was the seed for the development of the DNP degree.

There was a second report in 2005 from the National Academy of Sciences entitled *Advancing the Nation's Health Needs* (National Research Council Committee for Monitoring the Nation's Changing Needs for Biomedical, Behavioral, and Clinical Personnel, 2005) that impacted the decision to develop a practice-focused doctorate. This report called for the nursing profession to develop a nonresearch, clinical doctorate. This doctorate would serve to prepare expert practitioners who could also act as clinical faculty. The DNP-prepared nurse would fit the desired outcome of this report as well. Following these recommendations, nurses would have the opportunity to have a greater influence in all aspects of healthcare. The Affordable Care Act of 2010 began a transformation of the healthcare system in the United States. As the U.S. system moves into one of prevention, primary care, community health centers, and initiatives and quality of care, DNP-prepared nurses are well equipped to be on the forefront of this change. The education of DNP-prepared nurses, using the Essentials of DNP Education as the foundation, fits seamlessly into the new system as it is envisioned. The greatest opportunities for growth are found in the areas of leadership, preventative care, community and population health, advocacy for patients, and policy making and revision.

DNP-prepared nurses now have an opportunity to be on equal educational footing with other healthcare team professionals who have clinical doctorates. Currently, those professions and their credentials are the following:

Audiology	AuD
Pharmacy	PharmD
Physical Therapy	DPT
Psychology	PsyD or PsychD
Dentistry	DMD or DDS
Medicine	MD or DO

No longer will nurses be the least educated practitioner on the team, which often leads to an imbalance of power and influence. There are, however, some legal and professional barriers that impede nurses from moving forward as quickly as we would like or need to (Lathrop & Hodnicki, 2014). There are still legal restrictions in many states to APRN licenses, making it impossible to be able to fully practice independently. As of December, 2018, 22 states, plus the District of Columbia, have full practice and unrestricted licenses for NPs; 16 states have reduced practice licenses, which means that at least one aspect of care is limited or reduced legally and a career-long collaborative agreement is necessary with a medical doctor; and 12 states have restricted licenses in which at least one aspect of practice is restricted and career-long supervision is required for practice (American Association of Nurse Practitioners, 2018). This is a major stumbling block, and the IOM has called for full practice ability for all practitioners in order to be able to reach the goals set for patient and systems outcome (Altman, Butler, & Shern, 2016). If DNP-prepared nurses are going to make the contributions they are capable of, then full scope of practice needs to be put into place where it is not (Altman et al., 2016).

Another challenge is an unequal reimbursement scale for equal care. DNP-prepared APRNs need to be compensated equally with their medical doctor counterparts by organizations, insurance companies, and Medicare. Medicare reimburses services rendered by APRNs to residents of long-term care (LTC) facilities at a rate of 85% of a medical doctor. All APRNs, including DNP-prepared APRNs, need to advocate for this at the state and federal level by becoming politically active and donating funds to organizations that represent their needs.

Collaborative relationships can be another challenge faced by DNP-prepared APRNs due to interprofessional conflict (Keeling, 2009). The use of the "Doctor" or the prefix "Dr." by anyone other than an MD is being challenged by medical doctors. Some physicians see the expanding role of APRNs, and specifically the doctoral prepared DNP–APRN, as a threat and look to the legislative bodies to limit the scope of practice and the use of titles. Increased collaboration is necessary in first addressing these issues on a personal face-to-face basis and on the policy level as well.

A significant challenge to the DNP-prepared APRN exists within nursing itself. It is extremely bothersome that there is continued lack of support and in-fighting among ourselves about the value of the DNP degree and its comparison with the PhD degree or the people who hold these degrees. This does nothing for the presentation of a united front when fighting legislation, as outlined earlier.

This unfortunately is not a new phenomenon in nursing as we continue to question the need for a baccalaureate degree as the entry level to general practice. This conversation continues, despite the first ANA white paper on this subject being written in 1965—a full 54 years at the writing of this book! We are now debating the need, validity, and impact of the DNP degree in the same way rather than accepting it as a different but equal terminal degree (Beeber, Palmer, Waldrop, Lynn, & Jones, 2019). The challenge now is for those with the DNP degree to articulate their skills and their worth to the healthcare system, patients, and detractors alike. We need to be open to change and grow, with denigrating or devaluing something we are not part of. We need to be able to come together as one profession and support what each of us does and the path we chose to take to get there.

SUMMARY

The DNP-prepared nurse as a clinician was designed to be the pinnacle of the DNP degree, and many nurses chose this path. This chapter's goal was to outline the different specialties, certifications, and career options available with direct patient care. Although the chapter outlines a few of the challenges of the role, there are several counterpoints and advantages of the DNP-prepared nurse in direct patient care. The specialties and career options that are available are noteworthy and will serve as a guide for pursing the DNP degree and finding the best role to enhance professional growth.

REFLECTION QUESTIONS

1. What health trends were present that led to the development of the recommendation for APRNs to have a DNP degree as the entry level of education to practice?
2. What are some of the benefits of DNP education to the changing healthcare system?
3. What is your view of the added value of an APRN with an DNP degree over a master's-prepared APRN?

(*continued*)

(continued)

4. Are there any settings or roles in which a DNP-prepared APRN may be more prepared to work, or embody, than a master's-prepared APRN?
5. How well or poorly have we progressed in the IOM's vision for the future of nursing?
6. Reflect on the impact of medical doctors lobbying for legislation to limit the use of the title "Doctor" and the prefix "Dr." and limit the practice of APRNs.

References

Advanced Practice Registered Nurse Consensus Work Group and the National Council of State Boards of Nursing APRN Advisory Group. (2008). *Consensus model for APRN regulation: Licensure, accreditation, certification and education.* Retrieved from https://www.nursingworld .org/~4aa7d9/globalassets/certification/aprn_consensus_model_report_ 7-7-08.pdf

Altman, S. H., Butler, A. S., & Shern, L. (Eds.) (2016). *Assessing progress on the Institute of Medicine report* The Future of Nursing. Washington, DC: National Academies Press. Retrieved from https://www.ncbi.nlm.nih.gov/ books/NBK350160

American Association of Colleges of Nursing. (2004). *AACN position statement on the practice doctorate in nursing.* Retrieved from https://www .aacnnursing.org/Portals/42/News/Position-Statements/DNP.pdf

American Association of Colleges of Nursing. (2019). *Fact sheet: Doctor of nursing practice (DNP).* Retrieved from https://www.aacnnursing.org/ Portals/42/News/Factsheets/DNP-Factsheet.pdf

American Association of Nurse Practitioners. (2018). State practice environment. Retrieved from https://www.aanp.org/advocacy/state/state-practice -environment

American Midwifery Certification Board. (n.d.). *Why AMCB certification?* Retrieved from https://www.amcbmidwife.org/amcb-certification/why -amcb-certification-

Beeber, A. S., Palmer, C., Waldrop, J., Lynn, M. R., & Jones, C. B. (2019). The role of doctor of nursing practice-prepared nurses in practice settings. *Nursing Outlook, 67,* 354–364. doi:10.1016/j.outlook.2019.02.006

Campaign for Action. (2019). *Number of people receiving nursing doctoral degrees annually.* Retrieved from https://campaignforaction.org/resource/ number-people-receiving-nursing-doctoral-degrees-annually

DeCapua, M. (n.d.). *Guide to NP certification.* Retrieved from https://www
.nursepractitionerschools.com/faq/how-to-earn-np-certification

Doctor of Nursing Practice DNP. (n.d.). *BSN-DNP programs for BSN-prepared
nurses.* Retrieved from: https://www.doctorofnursingpracticednp.org/post
-bachelors-bsn-to-dnp-programs

Greiner, A., & Knebel, E. (Eds.). (2003). *Health professions education: A
bridge to quality.* Washington, DC: National Academies Press. Retrieved
from https://www.ncbi.nlm.nih.gov/books/NBK221528

Keeling, A. (2009). A brief history of advanced practice nursing in the United
States. In A. B. Hamric, J. A. Spross, & C. M. Hanson (Eds), *Advanced
practice nursing an integrative approach* (pp. 3–26). St. Louis, MO: Elsevier.

Kurtzman, E. T., & Barnow, B. S. (2017). A comparison of nurse practitioners, physician assistants and primary care physicians' patterns of practice and quality of care in health centers. *Medical Care, 55,* 615–622.
doi:10.1097/MLR.0000000000000689

Lathrop, B., & Hodnicki, D. R. (2014). The Affordable Care Act: Primary care
and the doctor of nursing practice. *Online Journal of Issues in Nursing, 19,* 7.
Retrieved from https://www.ncbi.nlm.nih.gov/pubmed/26824838

Laurant, M., van der Biezen, M., Wijers, N., Watananirum,K., Kontopantelis,
E., & van Vught, A. J. A. H. (2018). Nurses as substitutes for doctors in
primary care. *Cochrane Database of Systematic Reviews, 7,* CD001271.
doi:10.1002/14651858.cd001271.pub3

National Association of Clinical Nurse Specialists. (n.d.). *CNS competencies.*
Retrieved from https://nacns.org/professional-resources/practice-and
-cns-role/cns-competencies

National Association of Clinical Nurse Specialists. (2011). Clinical nurse specialist core competencies: Endorsing organations. Retrieved from https://
nacns.org/wp-content/uploads/2016/11/Endorsers.pdf

National Research Council Committee for Monitoring the Nation's
Changing Needs for Biomedical, Behavioral, and Clinical Personnel.
(2005). *Advancing the nation's health needs.* Washington, DC: National
Academies Press. Retrieved from https://www.ncbi.nlm.nih.gov/books/
NBK22622/pdf/Bookshelf_NBK22622.pdf

Patient Protection and Affordable Care Act, 42 U.S.C. § 18001 (2010).

RegisteredNurseRN.com. (n.d.). *CRNA program changes in 2025.* Retrieved
from https://www.registerednursern.com/crna-program-changes-in
-2025-dnap-vs-dnp-degree-to-become-a-crna/

Stanik-Hutt, J. (2008). Debunking the need to certify the DNP degree.
The Journal for Nurse Practitioners, 4, 739. doi:10.1016/j.murpra.2008
.09.009

Stanik-Hutt, J., Newhouse, R. P., White, K. M., Johantgen, M., Bass, E. B.,
Zangaro, G., … Weiner, J. P. (2013). The quality and effectiveness of care

provided by nurse practitioners. *The Journal for Nurse Practitioners, 9*, 492–500.e13. doi:10.1016/j.nurpra.2013.07.004

U.S. Bureau of Labor Statistics. (2019). *Occupational outlook handbook: Nurse anesthetists, nurse midwives, and nurse practitioners.* Retrieved from https://www.bls.gov/ooh/healthcare/nurse-anesthetists-nurse-midwives-and-nurse-practitioners.htm

6

The DNP-Prepared Nurse as an Executive

"Working in leadership roles in nursing requires a knowledge base in patient care, management, leadership, change theory, policies, finance, and information technology, to name a few. Most of this knowledge comes from experience working in different roles within nursing, unless you have a degree in nursing leadership or healthcare administration. However, the doctoral of nursing practice (DNP) prepares you for these types of roles. I hold a leadership position in a large academic medical center. This role requires guiding staff nurses through change, working with the interprofessional team to improve the workplace environment, and looking at the scope of nursing on a larger scale than the nursing unit. The academic curricula of the DNP teach us to look at healthcare and outcomes from a broader perspective. As a leader, how can we affect outcomes? The DNP degree has given me the tools to successfully lead change, engage staff in that change, effectively collaborate with a multidisciplinary team, and enhance/sustain that change through policy. I encourage nurses to take the leap and continue to advance with path to obtain a DNP; it will change your professional life."
—Kimberly Rivera, DNP, RN-BC, OCN

INTRODUCTION

The Nurse Executive

A nurse executive is a high-level professional administrator who works intensely behind the direct patient care scene to ensure that strategic goals align with the organization's mission. The nurse executive is a critical position, and the individual serves as role model for the organization. Frederickson and Nickitas (2011) identified the potential requirements to become a nurse executive, which include "minimum of a master's degree, at least 10 years' experience in administration and management with some level of experience with business, strategic and Magnet Recognition Program planning, as well as demonstrated collaborative, interpersonal skills with physicians and others members of the executive suite" (p. 345).

Nurse executives may also be identified with the following terminology:

- Nurse administrator
- Director of nursing
- Chief nursing officer/executive

A nurse executive is a member of senior leadership and ensures that the nursing staff has the resources and opportunities to provide and deliver the highest quality healthcare. The nurse executive is responsible for numerous daily functions in an organization, including the following:

- Monitoring nursing staff
- Implementing strategic goals
- Managing the organization's budget
- Instituting policies
- Collaborating with human resources
- Ensuring collective accountability
- Managing partnerships with healthcare providers and consumers
- Leading cost-effective patient care

LEADERSHIP: A COMMON THEME FOR DNP NURSES

A common thread throughout DNP programs and in practice is leadership. A fundamental question that often arises is: Is leadership innate or learned? This is a question that has multiple answers and

innate or learned? This is a question that has multiple answers and can be supported from several perspectives. The discussion of the origins of leadership is ongoing among professionals and the literature. The literature promotes advantages of each side of the question. Some individuals as early as in childhood can display leadership qualities. Many leaders have instincts to oversee units and projects, act as team leads, as well as possess the ability to motivate and encourage colleagues and patients. These leaders can be viewed as having natural talent.

Fast Facts

Leadership can be learned. One can learn from well-established leaders who can act as role models in the professional setting. Often, these leaders, having watched a director, chief nursing officer (CNO), manager, charge nurse, or even seasoned colleague, exhibit positive leadership skills that can be emulated. Good leaders motivate, support, guide, and can be instrumental in changing one's view of nursing and how he or she practices.

DNP programs promote leadership in the curriculum as well as in the development and implementation of the DNP project. Another important fact is that leadership skills can be applied to numerous situations in one's life (Box 6.1).

Mastering leadership skills in the professional arena is necessary for the DNP-prepared nurse executive. The DNP Essentials (American

BOX 6.1 LEADERSHIP SKILLS CAN BE APPLIED TO THE FOLLOWING SITUATIONS

1. Family
2. Relationships
3. Work
4. Professional

Association of Colleges of Nursing, 2006) have leadership skills and requirements embedded in each of them. Even though each Essential can clearly apply leadership concepts, the following Essentials are imperative to leading in order to evoke change within the healthcare arena.

1. Essential II: Organizational and Systems Leadership for Quality Improvement and Systems Thinking
2. Essential III: Clinical Scholarship and Analytical Methods for Evidence-Based Practice
3. Essential V: Health Care Policy for Advocacy in Health Care
4. Essential VI: Interprofessional Collaboration for Improving Patient and Population Health Outcomes
5. Essential VII: Clinical Prevention and Population Health for Improving the Nation's Health

The mastery of leadership skills for DNP students and DNP-prepared nurses, regardless of their stance on leadership being innate, learned, or a combination of the two, is a must. This is especially true for those DNP-prepared nurses who choose to occupy the role of a nurse executive. Guyton (2012) identified nine principles for successful leadership:

1. Commit to excellence
2. Measure the important issues
3. Build a culture around service
4. Create and develop leaders
5. Focus on employee satisfaction
6. Build individual accountability
7. Align behaviors with goals and values
8. Communicate on all levels
9. Recognize and reward success

These key concepts can be helpful for the DNP nurse executive and can be utilized in numerous situations, such as the following:

- Board meetings
- Staff meetings
- Research meetings
- Policy hearings
- Mentoring
- Collaboration with other healthcare providers and professionals

LEADERSHIP EXAMPLE

I had a nurse director who early on in my career posed one of the most important practice questions, and after 30 years, I still remember: "You need to learn to pick and choose your battles! Practice does not always follow a textbook; however, it is your responsibility as a nurse to do the best you can for your patients safely."

These words continue to replay in numerous daily encounters with colleagues, patients, and families, especially in today's healthcare environment. This leader has impacted my care delivery methods. She was an outstanding natural leader. She had the ability to motivate in a compassionate manner and was strong minded with excellent clinical skills. Her most impactful leadership qualities were that she was a realist and always supported nursing. Leaders supporting nurses regardless of the nursing role is imperative to successful leadership. I hope that each of you can reminisce about your important professional leader.

Beeber, Palmer, Waldrop, Lynn, and Jones (2019) performed a study examining the role of the DNP-prepared nurse in nursing administration. The results revealed that administrative and leadership roles were occupied with DNP-prepared nurses. The DNP nurse filled roles in several capacities, such as implementing improvement and quality projects, leading staffing initiatives, and reviewing and analyzing data for quality management. Bowie, DeSocio, and Swanson (2019) published a study examining the recent DNP-prepared nurses' current practice and application of DNP Essentials. The study acknowledged and supported the belief that DNP "education prepares advanced practice nurses for leadership across complex healthcare system" (p. 280).

ADMINISTRATIVE ROLES AND SETTINGS FOR THE DNP NURSE

DNP students often face a barrage of questions, such as why they are returning to schooling and what it will yield the individual, especially since many of the DNP students are already functioning as expert nurses. A good response is: "I don't know yet; there are too many options open to me." Options are numerous for a DNP-prepared nurse, especially within the confines of executive and administrative specialty.

Administrative roles for DNP-prepared nurses are not restricted to one option. The role of the nurse executive has a wide range of possibilities and often depends upon the stage of career, past experiences, and professional and personal goals. Administrative roles within the DNP scope can be different. *Administration* is a general term; however, administration and its relationship to nursing can be tailored to several practice roles. Beeber et al. (2019) identified that DNP nurses are satisfying the following two main administrative roles:

1. Administrative
   a. Managers
   b. Supervisors
   c. Primary and specialty healthcare practice administrators
2. Executive
   a. Chief nursing officers
   b. Healthcare systems executives and leaders

Fast Facts

Regardless of the official title, DNP-prepared nurses are being hired for key management and high-level leadership positions within the healthcare industry. In some instances, administrative roles are being created as organizations are understanding the value of the DNP nurse. This can be evidenced by the increase in job postings in various nursing outlets, with new and exciting executive/leadership position openings. This may be due to the ongoing mergers of smaller and larger organizations and health systems.

Administrative Role: Change in Focus

Currently, most organizations employ master's-prepared nurses in administrative and executive roles in the nursing arena. However, there is a high potential to see more DNP-prepared nurses applying for senior-level leadership positions, especially with the increased number of DNP programs and student enrollment.

Healthcare is continuing to evolve, and changes have already been seen in nursing leadership position requirements. In the 1990s, organizations encouraged and, in some cases, mandated nurse administrators and executives to pursue a master's degree, such as a master of science in nursing (MSN) or a master of business administration (MBA), or both. The rationale for organizations supporting nurse leaders to obtain an MBA was to meet the demands of the financial and business components associated with the ability to deliver complex and high-quality healthcare. Several universities across the nation were offering the dual MSN/MBA program. The concept of offering a dual master's degree was an innovative idea for leaders to deal with the changing healthcare environment; however, the literature identified that the number of students enrolling in dual MBA/MSN programs was relatively low. These combined programs faced significant challenges, such as indeterminate financial benefit to the student, available employment options, and increase in length of the program (Minnick, 1998).

Fast-forward almost 30 years, and the DNP-prepared nurse is an ideal candidate for meeting the complex and financially driven healthcare system. DNP-prepared nurses can blend leadership, finance, systems theory, patient care, and national health concerns, which makes them the best fit for administrative and executive roles. DNP-prepared nurses are fully equipped to fill these roles. A primary reason that the DNP-prepared nurse can be successful in the administrative track is because the DNP Essentials and curricula are designed to focus on the key components required to lead, such as the following:

- Leadership concepts
- Systems theory
- Analysis of data
- Identification of gaps in knowledge
- Health policy
- Critical thinking
- Mentoring
- Focus on quality and quality improvement
- Advanced clinical practice

DNP NURSES IN THE EXECUTIVE ROLE

As the number of nurses pursuing the DNP has increased, there has been an influx of nurse executives recognizing the potential benefits of the degree. Many nurse executives have identified the applicability of the DNP degree to their current role as a nurse executive. The literature supports the observation that those in the role of chief nursing officers/executives are pursuing the degree.

Lackey (2017) identified that CNOs who are looking toward retirement are enrolling in DNP programs; this indicates that CNOs are identifying the value of the DNP degree. In addition, CNOs who have successfully obtained the DNP degree can have firsthand knowledge of the potential impact of the DNP education, and they can embrace and support their nurses who are also planning for and completing the degree. Swanson and Stanton (2013) performed an interesting DNP capstone project to examine the perceptions of the DNP roles. The study concluded that the DNP is an "appropriate degree option for executive roles at aggregate, system and organizational levels." Beglinger (2016) also identified a variety of reasons the DNP degree is appealing to nurse executives:

- Challenging
- Lifelong learning
- Development of new knowledge
- Ability to participate by adding information to the literature
- Commitment to clinical scholarship
- Increased confidence

Nurse executives who are pursuing the DNP degree will have a solid understanding of the essentials and be able to create opportunities for their DNP-prepared nurses. Nurse executives and administrators are usually well seasoned and well versed in the following:

- National and state nursing requirements
- Current health policies
- Finances of the organization and healthcare environment
- Nursing and patient satisfaction
- Ability to implement change

Barry and Winter (2015) elegantly stated "of all the educational opportunities available today, the DNP Degree in Health System Leadership provides the optimum foundation for Chief Nurse Executives to lead within the current evolving healthcare industry. CNOs are prime candidates for obtaining the DNP degree and can be instrumental in making local and global changes to healthcare" (p. 528).

DNP LEADERSHIP ROLES WITHIN EVIDENCE-BASED PRACTICE AND RESEARCH DEPARTMENTS

Another area where DNP-prepared nurses are holding a seat and viewed as leaders is in research and evidence-based practice departments, councils, and committees. How nursing research is structured within the organization will determine the official title of the DNP nurse and the reporting plan. For example, some organizations, especially Magnet® hospitals, have an abundance of resources and have separate nursing research departments, advanced practice nurses departments, quality and improvement departments, and Magnet team/departments.

Some organizations may have nursing research and evidence-based practice projects generated from nursing education and/or another departments. Organizations may also have nurse research committees led by DNP nurses. For example, acute institutions that have the Magnet designation emphasize a shared governance model. In this model, staff nurses are the chairpersons of both units-based and hospital-wide committees, which focus on patient care. In addition to shared governance, staff nurses are encouraged to engage, produce, and implement evidence-based projects. DNP-prepared nurse administrators act as liaisons and mentors to the staff nurses in charge of the committees, providing recommendations and support. Yoder et al. (2014) revealed that it may be unrealistic for staff nurses to develop and implement evidence-based practice projects without the support of master's- or doctoral-prepared nurses who act as coaches, mentors, and champions.

Another area in which DNP-prepared nurses can occupy executive/leadership roles is in quality assurance departments. Quality improvement departments produce a significant amount of data and medical and nursing research, which DNP-prepared nurse can manage, analyze, and disseminate. Tussing et al. (2018) emphasized the importance of systems theory and how DNP nurses can guide and disseminate evidence and identify positive outcomes. In many organizations, especially Magnet-designated hospitals, staff nurses and advanced practice registered nurses are highly encouraged to participate and develop performance improvement projects, evidence-based practice projects, quality measures, and nursing research. Therefore, the literature and practice have determined that DNP-prepared nurses can be vital in assisting the nursing staff meet the demands and engage in evidence-based practice and research.

DNP LEADERSHIP ROLES FOR MAGNET PROGRAM DIRECTORS AND MAGNET SURVEYORS

Magnet designation can pose potential career opportunities for DNP-prepared nurses. Magnet is a national recognition designation that can be applied through the American Nursing Credentialing Center (ANCC). Magnet designation is an opportunity for organizations to showcase their professional nurses. Magnet requires the professional nurse to create, implement, and evaluate evidence-based practice projects in order to positively impact patient care. In addition, Magnet assesses how the nursing staff aligns with the organizationals goals. The Magnet Recognition Program was designed to serve as a road map to nursing excellence, which ultimately benefits the entire organization.

The Magnet Recognition Program also provides an avenue to support, promote, and emphasize the positive impact of the professional nurse via the following vehicles:

1. Career development
2. Nursing certification
3. Advanced education
4. Nursing research
5. Quality improvement
6. Patient outcomes

The media has played a vital role in identifying Magnet organizations, which is equated to Magnet nurses. Patients/customers recognize that the Magnet designation is known to promote higher quality care and better outcomes (ANCC, n.d.-b).

The Magnet recognition process has potential value and career opportunities for DNP-prepared nurses. It is not surprising that the DNP Essentials align nicely with the Magnet components (Table 6.1). For example, Lackey (2017) highlighted in a study that "Essential III of DNP education met a specific need identified for the magnet program director" (p. 304).

Table 6.1

Magnet Model Components and Related DNP Essentials

Magnet Model Components	Matching DNP Essentials
Transformational leadership	Essential II
	Essential VI
	Essential VII
Structural empowerment	Essential II
Exemplary professional practice	Essential I
	Essential VIII
New knowledge, innovation, and improvements	Essential II
	Essential III
	Essential IV
	Essential V
	Essential VI
Empirical quality results	Essential III

Therefore, the components aligning with the DNP Essentials, who better to occupy the roles of Magnet coordinators, Magnet directors, and Magnet surveyors?

These roles and function will vary depending on the organization's Magnet status and the organization's reporting structure. Lackey (2017) identified that DNP nurses are becoming Magnet program directors. The study revealed that the skill set is unique and "highly specialized" and that DNP nurses can pursue being Magnet directors. Although the author noted further research is needed, the connection between the Essentials and Magnet requirements can be a "good career path" for DNP-prepared nurses.

In practice, it has been observed that DNP-prepared nurses as well as PhD nurses have filled the Magnet directors and Magnet surveyor roles. Both the doctoral degrees produce nurses with excellent writing skills and the ability to analyze, interpret, and communicate data. In addition, DNP-prepared nurses have a concrete understanding of organizational systems, leadership, and current clinical requirements, which can allow for a successful and viable career path within the Magnet Recognition Program. There are other accrediting bodies such as the Joint Commission, which can also be a consideration for a DNP-prepared nurse's career options.

CERTIFICATION FOR THE ADMINISTRATIVE ROLE

Certification is a key factor in the DNP process; it allows DNP-prepared nurses to be updated and demonstrate excellence in their designated nursing fields. With that said, nursing certification is a personal preference. Each individual nurse must determine which is the most appropriate certification to hold based upon nursing specialty and career direction. The ANCC is a division of the American Nurses Association, which endorses nursing excellence in a global aspect through credentialing programs. Credentialing is also known as the "certification process." The ANCC offers numerous specialty certification opportunities for nurses in fields such as administration, staff development, family nurse, and adult and geriatric nurse practitioners, just to name a few. The certification identifies that the nurse has the advanced knowledge, ability, and understanding to provide safe quality care within the nursing specialty and is regarded highly within the organization and publicly (ANCC, n.d.-a).

It is important to understand that ANCC is one certification body, and there are numerous nursing specialty organizations that offer certifications, for example, Oncology Nursing Society, American Association of Critical Care Nurses, Holistic Nursing, and many others.

Fast Facts

Many nursing administrators and executives will hold a certification in Nursing Administration (Box 6.2). However, it is not uncommon for nurse administrators to have a dual or multiple certification. Many nurse leaders may decide to keep their specialty nursing organizations certification.

BOX 6.2   ANCC CERTIFICATION OPTIONS FOR NURSING ADMINISTRATORS

- **Nurse Executive Certification (NE-BC):** Available to licensed RNs who hold an MSN degree and have worked for

(continued)

BOX 6.2   ANCC CERTIFICATION OPTIONS FOR NURSING ADMINISTRATORS (*continued*)

a minimum of 24 months as a nurse manager, a supervisor, a director, or an administrator in the past 5 years.

■ **Nurse Executive Advanced Certification (NEA-BC):** Available to licensed RNs who have completed an MSN degree or a DNP degree and have worked for a minimum of 24 months as a nurse executive or the equivalent amount of time teaching nursing administration at the graduate level.

CHALLENGES FOR DNP NURSES IN THE ADMINISTRATIVE/EXECUTIVE ROLE

Challenges, obstacles, and/or barriers are inherent in every aspect of life. Although at times one may wish they do not exist, DNP-prepared nurses are not exempted. However, DNP-prepared nurses are equipped to navigate through the challenges. The most common challenges are as follows:

1. Defending the value of the DNP degree
   a. Working with other healthcare providers who do not understand the DNP role
   b. Role confusion
   c. Working with leaders who do not have a DNP degree
2. Determining the appropriate DNP role
   a. Finding the best matched role for career goals
   b. Employers developing roles for DNP nurses
3. Working in nontraditional nursing roles
   a. Transitioning to leadership positions
4. Dealing with financial issues and resources
   a. Staffing issues
   b. Cost of delivering care
      i. Complex patient care issues
      ii. Medicare and Medicaid
      iii. Health policy changes

   c. Organizations' available resources

   d. Reimbursement concerns

5. Working in a large healthcare system

   a. Managing a nursing unit

   b. Managing a nursing department/division

Fast Facts

Although challenges are encountered in every career, the DNP-prepared nurse has the education via the curriculum to embrace the challenges and have numerous employment opportunities within the administrative realm. DNP students can choose to pursue the capstone project within the administrative arena and add more knowledge to existing literature. The DNP Essentials can assist the DNP-prepared nurse in identifying problems, developing solutions, and providing high-quality care in a variety of leadership roles. Lastly, the DNP degree can provide an advantage in the job market when looking to change a career path toward an administrative role.

CONCLUSION

Future Directions

DNP programs and academic leadership need to contemplate developing a tracking method to determine how many DNP-prepared nurses practice in the administrative/executive roles. It would be beneficial to see the trends in the current market and the available career opportunities.

REFLECTION QUESTIONS

1. Have you worked with a leader who was instrumental in your career path or practice? Can you remember how that leader changed your practice?

(continued)

(continued)

2. What leadership skills do you possess? Do you believe the leadership skills are innate or learned?

3. Is an administrative role a potential career path for you? If so, why?

4. Do you currently work in an organization where a nurse executive/administrator, manager, or director holds a DNP degree and what is the culture related to DNP-prepared nurses?

5. Do you currently work in a Magnet-designated organization? If so, how does the DNP nurse function within the organization? If not, what is your belief regarding Magnet status?

6. Write a plan on how to mentor a staff nurse leading a nursing research council and development of an evidence-based practice project.

7. Identify challenges that a DNP nurse executive may encounter within your current organization and what solutions could be developed to overcome those challenges.

References

American Association of Colleges of Nursing. (2006). *The essentials of doctoral education for advanced nursing practice*. Retrieved from https://www.aacnnursing.org/Portals/42/Publications/DNPEssentials.pdf

American Nurses Credentialing Center. (n.d.-a). *About ANCC*. Retrieved from https://www.nursingworld.org/ancc/about-ancc

American Nurses Credentialing Center. (n.d.-b). *ANCC Magnet Recognition Program*®. Retrieved from https://www.nursingworld.org/organizational-programs/magnet

Barry, J., & Winter, J. (2015). Health system chief nurse executive: Is a DNP the degree of choice? *The Journal of Nursing Administration, 45,* 527–528. doi:10.1097/NNA.0000000000000255

Beeber, A., Palmer, C., Waldrop, J., Lynn, M., & Jones, C. (2019). The role of doctor of nursing practice-prepared nurses in practice settings. *Nursing Outlook, 67,* 354–364. doi:10.1016/j.outlook.2019.02.006

Beglinger, J. (2016). CNO's gearing up while many are winding down: The late career DNP. *Journal of Nursing Administration, 46,* 109–110. doi:10.1097/NNA.0000000000000305

Bowie, B., DeSocio, J., & Swanson, K. (2019). The DNP degree: Are we producing the graduates we intended? *Journal of Nursing Administration, 49,* 280–285. doi:10.1097/NNA.0000000000000751

Frederickson, K., & Nickitas, D. (2011). Chief nursing officer executive development: A crisis or a challenge? *Nursing Administrative Quarterly*, *35*, 344–353. doi:10.1097/NAQ.0b013e31822f8e5c

Guyton, N. (2012). Nine principles of successful nursing leadership. *American Nurse Today*. Retrieved from https://www.americannurse today.com/nine-principles-of-successful-nursing-leadership

Lackey, S. (2017). DNP preparation in supporting critical skills for Magnet® program directors. *Journal of Nursing Administration*, *47*, 303–304. doi:10.1097/NNA.0000000000000484

Minnick, A. (1998). Education in administration: Trends in MSN/MBA and MSN in nursing administration. *Journal of Nursing Administration*, *28*(4), 57–62.

Swanson, M., & Stanton M. (2013). Chief nursing officers' perceptions of the doctor of nursing practice degree. *Nursing Forum*, *48*, 35–44. doi:10.1111/ nuf.12003

Tussing, T., BrinkMan, B., Francis, D., Hixon, B., Labardee, R., & Chipps, E. (2018). The impact of the doctorate of nursing practice nurse in a hospital setting. *The Journal of Nursing Administration*, *48*(12), 600–602. doi:10.1097/NNA.0000000000000688

Yoder, L., Kirkley, D., McFall, D., Kirksey, K., StalBaum, A., & Sellers, D. (2014). CE: Original research staff nurses' use of research to facilitate evidence-based practice. *American Journal of Nursing*, *114*, 26–37. doi:10.1097/01 .NAJ.0000453753.00894.29

Further Reading

Nurse Practitioner Schools. (n.d.). *How do I become a nurse executive?* Retrieved from https://www.nursepractitionerschools.com/faq/how-to -become-nurse-executive

Nursing License Map. (n.d.). *Nurse executive*. Retrieved from https://nursing licensemap.com/advanced-practice-nursing/nurse-executive

7

The DNP-Prepared Nurse as an Educator

"Nurse educators combine knowledge and clinical expertise with a passion for teaching and learning. As a DNP nurse educator, I am responsible for preparing new nurses and advancing the development of practicing clinicians with the increasingly complex demands of today's healthcare system. The DNP curriculum provided an increased knowledge of informatics and healthcare technologies, quality improvement and safety, organizational and systems leadership, interprofessional collaboration for improving patient/population outcomes, and advocacy, as well as an advanced scientific and evidence-based approach for practice. As a DNP-prepared nursing professional, the contribution to nursing and healthcare includes the use of evidence-based practice, critical thinking and clinical decision-making, leadership, information technologies, and skilled communication in the classroom and in the clinical setting. As a DNP-prepared faculty member, I am committed to providing a rigorous academic and clinical education that combines different teaching/learning strategies that are adapted to student needs in order to prepare them to be confident and competent nursing professionals with the technical skills needed to be

successful and the knowledge that will improve the quality of patient care and outcomes. As a DNP-prepared nurse educator, I can successfully fulfill faculty obligations regarding teaching excellence, service, scholarship, and clinical practice."—Sharon Puchalski, DNP, APRN, WHNP-BC

INTRODUCTION

Foundations of the DNP in Education

The doctor of nursing practice (DNP) was initially proposed as a terminal degree in advanced practice nursing by the American Association of Colleges of Nursing (AACN, 2004). This was established to answer the call by industry in the form of the Institute of Medicine (IOM) and nurses alike for more advanced education of nurses who wished to remain firmly rooted in clinical expertise and scholarship. DNP-prepared nurses would gain the knowledge and credentials necessary to meet the needs of a more complex healthcare system and improve health outcomes for at-risk populations and the population at large. This then led to the development of the Essentials of Doctoral Education for Advanced Practice (AACN, 2006). These Essentials would be the building blocks to begin to inform the roles to be inhabited by nurses obtaining a DNP degree. One decision during this crucial time of the development phase of this new degree and the Essentials was to not include teaching expertise in the document. This was decided despite the fact that there was already a burgeoning nurse faculty shortage that was exhibiting no signs of abating in either the near or far off future. This fact significantly impacts the number of nurses in the United States, which is also at a critical point in history as the nursing shortage continues to grow. It was reported in the AACN's reports *Nursing Faculty Shortage Fact Sheet* (2017) and *Enrollment and Graduations in Baccalaureate and Graduate Programs in Nursing* (AACN's Institutional Data Systems and Research Center, 2019) that U.S. nursing schools turned down 75,029 qualified applicants due to four factors, including insufficient number of faculty members, which was the number one reason. In a separate AACN report entitled *Special Survey on Vacant Faculty Positions for Academic Year 2018–2019*

(Li, Turinetti, & Fang, 2018), it was revealed that there were 1,715 nursing faculty position vacancies across the country, with 85.8% of the respondents stating that not only there are vacant positions but also more positions and lines need to be added to attend to the students currently in the system. A total vacancy rate for faculty requiring or preferring a doctoral degree was estimated to be 7.9% nationally.

Nurse Education Quandary

Why or how this omission occurred is unclear. One possible reason is that nursing education is not always classified as "advanced practice," which is discussed later in this chapter. A second reason explored is that the task force given the task of developing the degree was made up solely of PhDs who believed that nursing education belongs solely in the purview of PhD-prepared nurses.

What we do know is that this one decision continues to have a negative effect on the hiring of nurses with earned DNP degrees into tenure-track positions in institutions of higher learning across the country (Agger, Oermann, & Lynch, 2014). The PhD-prepared nurse has historically been viewed as the only nurse who should be teaching in an academic setting. This can be traced to the movement of nursing educational programs from hospital-based training/diploma programs to university-based educational programs. This began in earnest in the 1950s as science and technology began to expand exponentially. The distinction of the PhD-prepared nurse being the only acceptable level of education for college and university faculty is tightly connected to the requirements of other disciplines, which are often nonclinical disciplines, and the university system of hiring and promotion. This currently accepted "truth" of hiring and promoting only PhD-prepared nurses for colleges and universities continues, often unchallenged, even though there are clear exceptions to this in other clinical disciplines such as doctor of pharmacy (PharmD), doctor of physical therapy (DPT), or doctor of medicine (MD).

Another point which is often not mentioned is that PhD-prepared nurses are similar to their DNP colleagues in their lack of formal education or coursework in the actual discipline of teaching, learning, and education as no coursework in those topics is included in either curriculum (Bullin, 2018). Therefore, in this particular area, having expertise in teaching and educating, the PhD and DNP graduates are similar.

Though not required for a teaching position, any nurse prepared at the doctoral level, both DNP and PhD, would need to engage in coursework specific to education and educational theory to be considered a competent educator (Kalb, 2008; Lewallen & Kohlenberg, 2011).

Another area of concern with the current PhD-educator/faculty model is the amount of time required to pursue their individual research area(s) of interest and the seeking of grant funds to support it. Little time is then left for student engagement and student-related activities (Bellini, McCauley, & Cusson, 2012).

Fast Facts

The responsibilities of research often force the PhD nurse to become far removed from clinical practice, which in today's healthcare arena is changing and accelerating at warped speed. This can lead to an increase in the disconnect between nursing education and the practice setting, which is one of the most common areas of complaints of service agencies employing new graduate nurses.

THE DNP NURSE AS EDUCATOR

The DNP-prepared nurse is firmly rooted in clinical practice and can play a vital role in changing the educational environment. Similar to the clinical DPT and PharmD, the DNP-prepared nurse educator can help alleviate the nursing faculty shortage, while bridging the gap the between practice and service (National Research Council's Committee for Mentoring the Nation's Changing Needs for Biomedical, Behavior, and Clinical Personnel, 2005).

DNP-prepared nurse educators naturally make the connection between practice and education that is lacking in today's healthcare system. This is especially true in light of the fact that teaching and education have always been included in the realm of nursing practice and care. However, some make the argument that teaching and education addressed in the nurse practice acts across the country and abroad is only in relation to patient teaching and patient education, not the education of future generations of nurses.

Roles and Settings

There are many roles a DNP-prepared nurse educator can inhabit in a number of different settings. The most common role and setting is that of an academician in an institution of higher learning. As nursing is an academic major found in many types of academic institutions, the role and responsibilities may be different based on what type of institution the DNP-prepared nurse educator is employed. See Table 7.1 for examples of these roles and settings.

There are also nonacademic settings where DNP-prepared nurse educators can find positions suiting their expertise and skills (Table 7.2). Some of these are large multihospital or multi-institution healthcare systems, acute care institutions, long-term care institutions, accrediting agencies, nurse consultant practices, and professional organizations. Some examples of the roles that may be found in some of these settings are as follows.

Table 7.1

DNP as Educator: Academic Roles and Settings	
Type of Institution	**DNP-Prepared Nurse Educational Roles**
Large research-focused university or college	■ Tenure track faculty ■ Nontenure track faculty ■ Clinical track faculty/nontenure ■ Adjunct faculty
Four-year college or university (with minimal to no funded research activity)	■ Nontenure track faculty ■ Clinical track faculty ■ Adjunct faculty ■ Tenure track faculty ■ Nontenure clinical faculty ■ Adjunct faculty
For-profit colleges and universities	■ Full-time faculty ■ Part-time faculty

Table 7.2

DNP as Educator: Nonacademic Roles and Settings

Setting	DNP-Prepared Nurse Educational Roles
Multihospital/institution systems; acute care institutions	■ VP/director/head/chair of nursing research or evidence-based practice ■ Corporate VP/director/head of nursing education ■ VP/director/head of nurse education ■ Unit/service-based nursing educator
Long-term care institutions	■ Corporate VP/director/head of nursing education ■ Institutional VP/director/head ■ Nurse educator
Nursing education consultant	■ Private practice that develops educational programs for clients ■ Educational systems analysis—needs assessments, program development, and evaluation

EDUCATIONAL CONSIDERATIONS

The controversies concerning DNP-prepared nurses as educators is apparent. In this section, we continue to explore the current state of DNP-prepared nurse educators related to their education. In light of the fact that the DNP degree was designed to increase the educational level of nurse practitioners (NPs), who are direct care providers, no formal educational courses are included in most program curriculum maps. This is also true of PhD programs across the country.

Fast Facts

There are some DNP programs in the United States that do offer a distinct nurse educator track. These specific schools are accredited by the National League for Nursing/National League for

(continued)

(*continued*)

Nursing Accrediting Commission (NLN/NLNAC), not the American Association of Colleges of Nursing/Commission on Collegiate Nursing Education (AACN/CCNE). The AACN/CCNE does not recognize nurse education as an advanced practice role and therefore will not accredit DNP programs with this formal track (Wittman-Price, Waite, & Woda, 2017).

The AACN's Futures Task Force report (2015) added more confusion to the growing DNP-prepared nurse educator debate. It stated in the clarifying statement that PhD in nursing was primarily research training for nurse scientists, not preparation for the role of faculty. In the same report, the AACN stated that DNP-prepared nurse educators should seek additional coursework in educational theory and practice but did not make the same recommendation for PhD-prepared nurses entering academia (AACN, 2015). This is a curious statement given that the majority of neither program includes education-specific coursework or practice. No explanation has yet been offered for this dichotomy of these statements. Both PhD-prepared and DNP-prepared nurses should be seen as viable candidates for teaching at the college level for both tenure and nontenure lines.

Despite the fact that there are only a small number of schools that offer a DNP degree in nursing education, graduates of DNP programs are joining the faculty ranks in significant numbers. One study examined the labor impact of DNP graduates by surveying 1,308 DNP-prepared nurses (Minnick, Kleinpell, & Allison, 2019). The top three titles reported by the respondents as being their end employment goal were NP (34%), certified registered nurse anesthetist (26.9%), and nurse educator, such as dean, director, faculty, continuing education coordinator, or hospital-based nursing educator (17%; Minnick et al., 2019). Clearly, DNP-prepared nurses and institutions across the country are recognizing the DNP degree as an appropriate terminal degree for nurse educators.

One reason for this may be the lack of acceptance of the role of nurse educator as an advanced practice role. The first change that needs to be made for nursing education to be viewed as advanced practice is to view it as a part of nursing practice and not a separate and distinct entity somehow removed from practice. Nursing is a practice-based profession, and therefore, it follows a logical order that expert practitioners should be involved with the education of new nurses, as well as nurses seeking specialty education at the master's level.

One way of countering the concern about DNP-prepared nurses not being prepared for the role of faculty would be to include educational courses with the curricula (Agger et al., 2014; Box 7.1). It would stand to reason that if this should become the norm in the future, it should also be required of PhD programs. Another measure that could be instituted is the evaluation of competencies related to teaching for all who teach regardless of degrees.

BOX 7.1   COURSES REQUIRED FOR A CAREER IN NURSE EDUCATION

Curriculum development/design
Role of the nurse educator
Program assessment/evaluation
Classroom teaching strategies
Educational technology

Pedagogy of teaching
Adult learning theory
Student assessment/evaluation
Clinical teaching strategies
Legal aspects of education

CERTIFICATIONS

The AACN Essentials of Doctoral Education for advanced nursing practice states "[a]ll DNP graduates, prepared as APNs, must be prepared to sit for national specialty APN certification" (2006, p. 17). This statement from the AACN implies there could be DNP-prepared nurses who are not prepared as APRNs as only those prepared as APRNs need to be certified. It should also be noted that the concept was put forth early in the development of DNP programs. It seems to acknowledge that despite the original-stated intent of the degree being developed and designed for the traditionally accepted APRN roles, that either room was left for, or it was anticipated, that nurses who wanted nontraditional APRN roles may in fact be drawn to a practice-based doctorate as opposed to a research doctorate. The certifications accepted by the *Consensus Model for APRN Regulation: Licensure, Accreditation, Certification & Education* (APRN Consensus Work Group & the National Council of State Boards of Nursing [NCSBN] APRN Advisory Committee, 2008) are listed in Table 7.3.

Table 7.3

Nursing Certifications Accepted by the Consensus Model for APRN Regulation

American Nurses Credentialing Center (ANCC)

Adult gerontology, acute care	AGACNP-BC
Adult gerontology, primary care	AGPCNP-BC
Family	FNP-BC
Psychiatric mental health	PMHNP-BC

Pediatric Nursing Certification Board (PNCB)

Pediatric, primary care	CPNP-PC
Pediatric, acute care	CPNP-AC

National Certification Corporation (NCC)

Neonatal	NNP-BC
Women's health gender related	WHNP-BC

American Academy of Nurse Practitioners Certification Program (AANPCP)

Family	FNP-C
Adult gerontology, primary care	NP-C or ANP-
Emergency	ENP-C

American Association of Critical Care Nurses (AACCN)

Adult gerontology, acute	ACNPC-AG

American Association of Nurse Anesthetists (AANA)

Certified registered nurse anesthetist	CRNA

American College of Nurse Midwives (ACNM)

Certified nurse midwife	CNM

Source: Data from Advanced Practice Registered Nurse Consensus Work Group & the National Council of State Boards of Nursing APRN Advisory Committee. (2008). *Consensus model for APRN regulation: Licensure, accreditation, certification & education.* Retrieved from https://www.aacn.org/~/media/aacn-website/nursing-excellence/standards/aprnregulation.pdf?la=en

THE ADVANCED PRACTICE ROLE

The next logical question that needs to flow from this implication has to be: Are there other advanced roles in nursing that are, or should be, considered advanced practice nursing roles? Advanced practice roles such as nurse educator, nurse informaticist, public health nurse, and nurse administrator are all roles that require advanced education but have historically been separated out from direct care roles as not being "practice." This separation occurs despite the fact that nurses in these roles have the ability to have a more positive, global influence on patient outcomes and nursing as a profession. It is time to stop separating nurses and consider us a whole profession, based in practice, with multiple facets of practice.

Another certification relative to nurse educators, regardless of educational preparation (master's, DNP, or PhD) is the Certified Nurse Educator (CNE) exam administered by the NLN. This has been the certification exam for the specialty of nurse educators. It is an exam that is accredited by the National Commission for Certifying Agencies (NCAA), the accrediting body of the National Organization for Competency Assurance (NLN, n.d.). This accreditation demonstrated that the CNE exam is in compliance with the NCAA standards for the Accreditation of Certification Programs. This level of standardization is indicative of the validity of the exam and the expertise of the educator who holds this credential. The ANA made a statement that certification was not necessary for advanced specialties that did not have direct care as their primary focus (Wittman-Price et al., 2017). This is an interesting statement because it is unusual for a professional body to discourage its member from being certified as it is often seen as a positive and valuable asset. Despite the statement, the NLN continues to offer the exam. In fact, it offers two nurse education certifications: one is the CNE for faculty who teach in the academic classroom setting and the other certifies academic clinical nurse educators. In the online overview of the CNE exam on the NLN website, the rationale for creating the exam was to "[establish] nursing education as a specialty area of practice and [create] a means for faculty to demonstrate their expertise in their role" (NLN, n.d., "Value of Certification").

Another form of certification is a DNP certification exam, which is required by some programs that are based on physician competencies.

The exam has been drawn from questions taken from the U.S. Medical Licensing Exam Step 3 (Stanik-Hutt, 2008). Fortunately, the use of the exam has not been adopted by a majority of the programs currently accepting students and is not widespread. It does not address any aspect of the nursing advanced practice role and can be seen as furthering the divide between physicians and APRNs rather than working toward a partnership built on our individual strengths and skill sets. There has been a great deal of discussion concerning the standardized certification of DNP-prepared nurses. To further support the point of view that developing a certification exam is not necessary or desired, the Nurse Practitioner Roundtable (NPR), a coalition of various NP professional organizations, put forth a statement. The statement was that academic degrees are earned by successfully completing a course of study and that any certification exam would be too broad to be meaningful (Nurse Practitioner Roundtable, 2008).

Fast Facts

Currently, the only requirement for DNP certification is the individual APRN specialty. For all those who function in the role of a nurse educator, DNP or PhD, full time or part-time, the CNE or CNEcl are the only certifications available to validate expertise. Both are currently voluntary.

CHALLENGES AND OPPORTUNITIES

In the case of the DNP-prepared nurse educators, as is often the case with many things in life, the challenges of a situation also present the opportunities. One of the first challenges for this particular role is the identification of nursing education as a practice-based specialty. Currently, there are only four roles designated as advanced practice roles according to the *Consensus Model for APRN Regulation: Licensure, Accreditation, Certification & Education* (APRN Consensus Work Group & the NCSBN APRN Advisory Committee, 2008).

1. Certified nurse specialist
2. Certified nurse midwife

3. Certified NP
4. Certified registered nurse anesthetist (APRN Consensus Work Group & the NCSBN APRN Advisory Committee, 2008)

Part of the argument for not including nursing education or any of the other preceding specialties is that no additional licensing or certification is necessary for teaching nursing but only an advanced academic degree (Alexander & Emerson, 2011). However, the counterpoint to that way of thinking about other specialties is that nurse educators in academic and clinical settings impact patient health outcomes through the preparation of new nurses, which is in keeping with the definition of advanced practice (Alexander & Emerson, 2011). We need to stop treating nursing education as a separate entity from practice as they are integrally connected to one another.

Nurse educators use various strategies both in the classroom and in the clinical area to assist in the development of new nurses. Nursing education is dynamic to meet the needs of students with various learning styles, entering an ever-changing, complex healthcare system. We need to begin to expand our definition of "practice" to include nurse educators, administrators, and others as we have expanded out the definition of clinical experiences to include simulation (Wittman-Price et al., 2017). This expanded definition then easily allows the inclusion of DNP-prepared educators as APRNs.

Closely following this first challenge is a second one that may be more complicated because it does not just involve nurses changing how nurses think; it involves changing minds and systems. The first part of this challenge is the discussion about whether or not DNP-prepared nurses be hired as faculty in colleges and universities. The next part of the challenge is, if the answer is yes, should they be hired as faculty; then should they be hired into tenure track lines or be delegated to only a lower level of the academic hierarchy—a non-tenure position? The last part of the challenge is the systems part of the equation: If hired into a tenure track, would the DNP-prepared nurse educator be able to meet the requirements for promotion? We believe strongly that the answer to all three parts of this challenge is a resounding yes!

One point of support of this opinion is that this is already successfully occurring in many institutions in the United States, and what change needs to be made for uniform acceptance of this new paradigm in nursing education remains a question. It is not however a new concept to all of education. Other practice-based disciplines, such as DPT, PharmD, and audiologist (AuD), all have faculty members who occupy tenure track lines and get promoted. The precedent already exists; it is up to us as nurses to open our minds to a new concept. One of the ongoing arguments against the DNP-prepared nurse educator in tenure track positions has been the perception that they should/would not be eligible for tenure because they are not educated to perform original research due to their practice focus.

The first point to argue against this is that some programs do require original research as part of the capstone project of evidence-based practice, though not all. The system used by many colleges and universities for promotion and tenure is the Boyer Model of Scholarship (Bellini et al., 2012; Stark, 1996; Zychowicz & Meleis, 2011). It has been argued that the DNP-prepared nurses, with their focus squarely in practice, would not meet the requirements of scholarship required for tenure appointment as determined in the Boyer model. However, there have been a number of examples provided in the literature that point to the congruence between DNP competencies and Boyer's Scholarship Model and definition (Bellini et al., 2012; Dreher, Clinton, & Sperhac, 2014; Trautman, Idzik, Hammersla, & Rosseter, 2018).

In this time of a crucial nursing shortage, that is on track to continue to worsen, and a nursing faculty shortage that is also widening and impacting the number of nurses in the work-force, DNP-prepared nurse educators could more than adequately fill some of these positions, both tenured and nontenured (Agger et al., 2014; Danzey et al., 2011; Dreher et al., 2014; Feldman, Greenberg, Jaffe-Ruiz, Kaufman, & Cignarale, 2015; Hammatt & Nies, 2015; Minnick et al., 2019).

As the enrollment in DNP programs continues to increase, there will be a greater need for faculty for these programs who can teach these students—PhD-prepared nurses who are not familiar with DNP competencies and certified APRNs with no doctoral education but direct care expertise. As indicated in the survey by Minnick et al. (2019), DNP-prepared nurses choosing the educational role are only third behind NPs and certified registered nurse anesthetists, and the trend is expected to continue with more DNP-prepared nurses looking to join the academic ranks. Schools of nursing are going to have make critical decisions about how to proceed. Will they choose to stay with a narrow view of scholarship? And who should be teaching future nurses? Or will they choose to be open, to broaden definitions of practice, scholarship, and advanced practice to meet the health needs of the global population by integrally linking scholarship and practice?

CONCLUSION

This chapter has presented some of our bigger challenges as we move into a new era of an increasing number of DNP-prepared nurses and specifically those choosing nursing education as their setting. It is up to us to make these challenges our opportunities.

REFLECTION QUESTIONS

1. Do you view nursing education as nursing practice? Why, or why not?
2. Are excellent practitioners always the best choice as educators?
3. Should nurses who assume the role of nursing educator be required to take formal educational coursework? If yes, DNP, PhD, MSN, or all of them? Why, or why not?
4. Should DNP-prepared nurse faculty be eligible for tenure?
5. In the capacity of a tenured faculty, research is often a requirement. Should DNP-prepared faculty be expected to conduct original research?
6. If it is decided that DNP-prepared nurses should not perform research, what other academic or practice activities could or should be substituted for the tenure process?
7. Should there be umbrella certification for the DNP degree, or is the specialty certification sufficient?

References

Advanced Practice Registered Nurse Consensus Work Group & the National Council of State Boards of Nursing APRN Advisory Committee. (2008). *Consensus model for APRN regulation: Licensure, accreditation, certification & education.* Retrieved from https://www.aacn.org/~/media/aacn -website/nursing-excellence/standards/aprnregulation.pdf?la=en

Agger, C. A., Oermann, M. H., & Lynn, M. R. (2014). Hiring and incorporating doctor of nursing practice-prepared nurse faculty into academic nursing programs. *Journal of Nursing Education, 53*, 439–446. doi:10.3928/01484834-20140724-03

Alexander, M., & Emerson, E. (2011). Point counterpoint: Is nursing education considered an advanced practice role? *The Journal of Nurse Practitioners, 7*, 370–371. doi:10.1016/j.nurpra.2011.03.028

American Association of Colleges of Nursing. (2004). *AACN position statement on the practice doctorate in nursing.* Retrieved from https://www.aacnnursing.org/Portals/42/News/Position-Statements/DNP.pdf

American Association of Colleges of Nursing. (2006). *The essentials of doctoral education for advanced nursing practice.* Retrieved from https://www.aacnnursing.org/Portals/42/Publications/DNPEssentials.pdf

American Association of Colleges of Nursing. (2015). *Futures task force—Final report.* Retrieved from http://www.aacnnursing.org/Portals/42/Downloads/Futures/Futures-Task-Force-Final-Report.pdf

American Association of Colleges of Nursing. (2017). *Nursing faculty shortage fact sheet.* Retrieved from http://www.aacnnursing.org/portals/42/news/factsheets/faculty-shortage-factsheet-2017.pdf

American Association of Colleges of Nursing's Institutional Data Systems and Research Center. (2019). *2018–2019 enrollment and graduations in baccalaureate and graduate programs in nursing.* Washington, DC: Author.

Bellini, S., McCauley, P., & Cusson, R. M. (2012). The doctor of nursing practice graduate as faculty member. *Nursing Clinics of North America, 47*, 547–556. doi:10.1016/j.cnur.2012.07.0004

Bullin, C. (2018). To what extent has doctoral (PhD) education supported academic nurse educators in their teaching roles: An integrative review. *BMC Nursing, 17*(6). doi:10.1186/s12912-018-0273-3

Danzey, I. M., Emerson, E., Fitzpatrick, J. J., Garbutt, S. J., Rafferty, M., & Zychowicz, M. E. (2011). The doctor of nursing practice and nursing education: Highlights, potential and promise. *Journal of Professional Nursing, 27*, 311–314. doi:10.1016/j.profnurs.2011.06.008

Dreher, M. C., Clinton, P., & Sperhac, A. (2013). Can the Institute of Medicine trump the dominant logic of nursing? Leading the change in advanced practice education. *Journal of Professional Nursing, 30*, 104–109. doi:10.1016/j/profnurs.2013.09.004

Feldman, H. R., Greenberg, M. J., Jaffe-Ruiz, M., Kaufman, S. R., & Cignarale, S. (2015). Hitting the nursing faculty shortage head on: Strategies to recruit, retain, and develop nursing faculty. *Journal of Professional Nursing, 31*, 170–178. doi:10.1016/j.profnurs.2015.01.007

Hammatt, J. S., & Nies, M. A. (2015). DNP's: What can we expect? *Nurse Leader, 13*, 64–66. doi:10.1016/j.mnl.2015.03.014

Kalb, K. (2008). Core competencies of nurse educators: Inspiring excellence in nurse educator practice. *Nursing Education Perspectives*, *29*, 217–219. Retrieved from https://journals.lww.com/neponline/Abstract/2008/07000/Core_Competencies_of_Nurse_Educators__Inspiring.13.aspx

Lewallen, L. P., & Kohlenberg, E. (2011). Preparing the nurse scientist for academia and industry. *Nursing Education Perspective*, *32*, 22–25. doi:10.5480/1536-5026-32.1.22

Li, Y., Turinetti, M., & Fang, D. (2018). Special survey on vacant faculty positions for academic year 2018–2019. Retrieved from https://www.aacnnursing.org/Portals/42/News/Surveys-Data/Vacancy18.pdf

Minnick, A. F., Kleinpell, R., & Allison, T. L. (2019). DNP's labor participation, activities, and reports of degree contributions. *Nurse Outlook*, *67*, 89–100. doi:10.1016/j.outlook.2018.10.008

National League for Nursing. (n.d.). *Certification for nurse educators*. Retrieved from http://www.nln.org/Certification-for-Nurse-Educators

National Research Council's Committee for Mentoring the Nation's Changing Needs for Biomedical, Behavior, and Clinical Personnel. (2005). *Advancing the nation's health needs*. Washington, DC: National Academies Press. Retrieved from https://researchtraining.nih.gov/sites/default/files/pdf/nas_report_2005.pdf

Nurse Practitioner Roundtable. (2008, June). *Nurse practitioner DNP education, certification and titling: A unified statement*. Washington, DC: Author. Retrieved from https://www.pncb.org/sites/default/files/2017-02/DNP_Unified_Statement.pdf

Stanik-Hutt, J. (2008). Debunking the need to certify the DNP degree. *The Journal for Nurse Practitioners*, *4*(10), 739. doi:10.1016/j.nurpra.2008.09.009

Stark, P. L. (1996). Boyer's multidimensional nature of scholarship: A new framework for schools of nursing. *Journal of Professional Nursing*, *12*, 268–276. doi:10.1016/S8755-7223(96)80006-8

Trautman, D. E., Idzik, S., Hammersla, M., & Rosseter, R. (2018). Advancing scholarship through translational research: The role of PhD and DNP prepared nurses. *Online Journal of Issues in Nursing*, *23*. doi:10.3912/OJIN.Vol23No02Man02

Wittman-Price, R., Waite, R., & Woda, D. L. (2017). The role of the educator. In H. M. Dreher & M. E. S. Glasgow (Eds.), *Role development for doctoral advanced nursing practice* (pp. 181–197). New York, NY: Springer Publishing Company.

Zychowicz, M. E., & Meleis, A. J. (2011). Point counterpoint: Should DNP's occupy tenured faculty positions. *The Journal of Nurse Practitioners*, *7*, 280–281. doi:10.1016/j.nurpra.2011.02.013

8

The DNP-Prepared Nurse as an Informatics Specialist

"My first experience with computers in the healthcare setting was in the 1970s. A very basic system was used to register for continuing education courses. This was at an academic medical center in New England. I was fascinated by the fact that I could select from a list of courses and register electronically. Even more amazing was the fact that for each course I selected, my name would appear in the response: 'Thank you, Teresa, for registering for this course.' I had no prior experience with computers, and it was enthralling to see my name on the screen.

In the 1980s at a medical center in California, I had my next experience with a registration system for patients. I could immediately see the benefits of this electronic system. I could see pending transfers into our unit in real time. As a charge nurse, this was a great help in planning assignments and care. Then, in the 1990s, I was involved in the implementation of a clinical information system. It was basic order entry for lab tests; however, I immediately saw the benefit to patients and nursing.

As I explored what computerization would mean to the nursing profession, I realized that I needed to enhance my skills and education. I anticipated that nurses would need to incorporate the computer into their day to day workflow. Therefore, I focused on the clinical applications and participated in the implementation of the order entry system. At the same time, I began my journey for a DNP. When I completed my DNP program, the DNP degree was in its infancy.

I was progressing in clinical informatics in an acute care facility in northern New Jersey. I was initially hired into a 'temporary' position for the implementation of the order entry system. This concerned me because I was unsure if I would have a position after 1½ years. Twenty years later, I was the administrative director in information technology for clinical systems. I directed a multidisciplinary team comprised of nurses, pharmacists, respiratory therapists, nutritionists, radiology techs, and clinical analysts. My role incorporated nursing science, computer science, and information science. I needed to consider communication theory and change management theory as they relate to all aspects of clinical system implementation. My DNP education provided both the core sciences and theoretical concepts. The two key concepts that have allowed over 30 years of DNP informatics role success are:

1. Remember, there is always a patient at the end of every transaction.
2. Design a system that can be used by every clinician, especially the one who is caring for the patient at 2 a.m. in the morning with minimal IT support. Make it work for them!"—Theresa Moore, DNP, RN-BC, NE-BC, CPHIMS

INTRODUCTION

The Journey of Informatics

Computers in healthcare have been available since the 1960s. The first systems used in healthcare were primarily financial systems used for registration and billing. Nurses use these systems for admission, discharge, and transfer functions. As computer systems became more integrated into healthcare, a gap was identified. Clinicians needed to take advantage of technology to care for patients. Therefore, the need for the development of clinical applications was necessary. The functions in these clinical systems included processing orders, administering medications, and clinical documentation. These were some of the first applications implemented in healthcare. During the early implementations, very few nurses were working with information technology (IT) staff. The results were systems that were not intuitive to clinical staff. Administrators recognized this deficiency and began to hire nurses in specific roles for the implementation of clinical applications.

Fast Facts

Nursing informatics was first identified as a specialty by the American Nurses Association (ANA) in 1992. *"Nursing informatics (NI)* is the specialty that integrates nursing science with multiple information management and analytical sciences to identify, define, manage, and communicate data, information, knowledge, and wisdom in nursing practice. NI supports nurses, consumers, patients, the interprofessional healthcare team, and other stakeholders in their decision-making in all roles and settings to achieve desired outcomes. This support is accomplished using information structures, information processes, and information technology" (ANA, 2015, p. 1).

As computer systems became more pervasive in the healthcare field, informatics experts were needed to facilitate system implementation. It was necessary to integrate computers into the workflow of nurses and healthcare providers. Computer systems needed to be intuitive, safe, and seamlessly integrated into the day-to-day activities of patient care. Nurses needed to be involved in every step of the system life cycle, which includes the following:

1. Selection design
2. Testing
3. Education
4. Implementation
5. Issue resolution
6. Maintenance

Involvement needed to occur at all levels—all levels of the cycle and all levels of clinical staff. Nursing supports the successful integration of applications. The challenge for this was to enhance user experiences with information systems (Hassett, 2006). Hassett (2006) defines the work that was done to facilitate the integration. Nurses were active participants in defining practice environment and education. Nurses acquired a new body of knowledge related to information systems.

Process of System Selection

The doctor of nursing practice (DNP)-informatics specialist as a project director would oversee the integrated testing. Crucial to the integration is education of the staff on the new workflow, the initial step for system selection; the chief nursing informatics officer (CNIO) participates in vendor demonstrations and site visits. For system design, staff nurses are recruited to identify current workflow, proposed new workflow, and impact analysis. Working as clinical analysts and in collaboration with system analysts, nurses become the heart, eyes, and ears of the system. New and existing policies are threaded through the design of the system. Included in this are organizational, state, and federal policies related to healthcare IT.

Testing of the newly designed system is accomplished at many levels. Unit testing allows the staff nurse to determine usability and accuracy as related to the organization's workflow. Integrated testing allows for a more complex assessment of the new system and how it interacts with other components of the system or legacy systems.

Education is one of the most important components of system implementation. Nursing and clinical staff must be properly educated on all aspects of the new system. Education should focus not just on the screens and new features but also on how the nurse would care for patients utilizing the new system. New policies need to be highlighted during the educational process.

The actual implementation or "go-live" requires support from the C-Suite, which includes the following (however, the CNIO leads the team):

1. Chief nursing officer
2. Chief operating officer
3. Chief executive officer
4. Chief financial officer

The go-live is a carefully orchestrated plan that details every step of the implementation of a computer system. The key components in this plan include scheduling of super users and support staff, IT staff, and clinical and nursing informatics staff at the direction of the project director. The timeline covers preimplementation tasks through resolution of system, training, and staffing issues.

Informatics Resolution

Issue resolution is similar to the triaging of patients in the emergency room. Issues are identified and logged by numerous healthcare provider support staff. The issue log is then reviewed by the DNP and IT project directors. The issues are prioritized based upon urgency and safety. Any issue that is classified as an enhancement is given a lower priority. Issues related to medication administration, order entry, and documentation are ranked based upon their need. A team of clinical and system analysts works to resolve the issue as quickly as possible. Once the urgent and emergent issues are resolved, the system can transition to maintenance.

The DNP project director is responsible, in collaboration with the IT project director, to prioritize the maintenance of the system. Enhancements are reviewed and ranked by priority. The project directors then reassess the team resources to determine those who will transition to maintenance or education.

ROLES AND SETTINGS FOR THE INFORMATICS SPECIALIST

DNP Informatics Specialist as CNIO

According to the American Organization of Nursing Leadership (AONL), a new type of nursing leader has emerged. This leader role is titled "Nursing Informatics Executive," also known as "the CNIO." The implementation of the electronic health record (EHR) with electronic documentation was key in the development of this role. The nursing informatics executive holds a minimum degree at the master's level and preferably at the doctoral level (American Organization of Nurse Executives, 2012). The AONL further identifies the workflow that redesigns incorporating safety, quality, and efficiency, guided by the nursing informatics executive, that will help to bridge practice education and research.

For the CNIO to excel, certain skills and knowledge are necessary. Hassett (2006) defined the following:

1. Primary driver for organizing the process
2. Providing strategic and business objectives and planning
3. Understanding the mission, vision, and value of the organization
4. Alignment of organization goals
5. Identification of quality improvement metrics
6. Collaborating with business and administrative executives to ensure system integration and maximization
7. Using technology for positive change in the budget, resource allocation, workflow reengineering, employee satisfaction, productivity, and revenue
8. Ensuring all stakeholders are at the table and overseeing the completion of documentation such as functional assessments, system requirements, and request for proposal
9. Implementing real-time alerts for both compliance and safety; storing data appropriately so that they are retrievable in both concurrent and retrospective manners
10. Identifying and approving system reports, analytics, data definitions, nomenclature, workflow, and rules associated with the system

Communication and Change Management

Communication and change management theory also play an important part. Change management will assure the quality and safety during the transition process. The change management function is to enhance efficiency by providing a seamless transition to the new clinical system. This includes data conversion and ensuring clinical needs occur without adversely impacting scope and resources. Communication plans must be developed and implemented. The change management process includes the adequate distribution of hardware for clinical staff and appropriate education as needed on the hardware.

The CNIO is the executive in charge of delivery, direction, and governance of clinical system implementation, providing guidance to all advisory groups, including the clinical advisory group and the executive advisory group. Chairs of the *clinical advisory group* include the chief nursing officer, the chief medical officer, and the chief medical information officer. Members include representatives from compliance, medical departments, and patient care including nursing, pharmacy, respiratory, ambulatory, and other interdisciplinary departments.

The *executive advisory group* is chaired by patient safety, finance, and performance improvement. Members of the executive advisory group include operations, health information management, and organizational education. These two groups oversee the direction of the implementation.

The teams responsible for project delivery are under the direction of the clinical project director, the chief technical officer, and the financial project director. Members of the *delivery team* include project coordinators for each specific team and members from interdisciplinary departments. These teams focus on clinical specialties such as the emergency department, pharmacy, ancillary departments, reporting and health information, interfaces, and ambulatory.

The *governance committee* includes members of the C-Suite and senior leadership. This committee provides input to the project executive to ensure alignment with organizational and strategic goals. The CNIO as project executive provides periodic updates to the committee at a macro level. The purpose is to ensure that the project remains on target and within budget. This is a high-level oversight to ensure goals are met.

At the direction level, the project executive ensures that milestones within each project plan are met. Details of the budget and the project plan are reviewed at this level; input from above and below are incorporated into meetings for the direction group. At the delivery level, input is provided from stakeholders and staff up to the project directors. Project directors then bring this information to the project executive. The flow of information occurs up and down committee structures. Pulling all this together is the project executive. The EHR project structure is detailed in Figure 8.1.

Fast Facts

The CNIO provides direction and professional support in the selection, design, implementation, and maintenance of computerized information systems; the role utilizes the informatics tools of IT,

(continued)

(continued)

information structures, and information management and communication. Nursing data are processed into information and knowledge to support the practice of nursing and the delivery of patient care, all aligned with organizational goals. The CNIO has expert clinical and IT knowledge and applies best practice to the management of the clinical information system lifecycle.

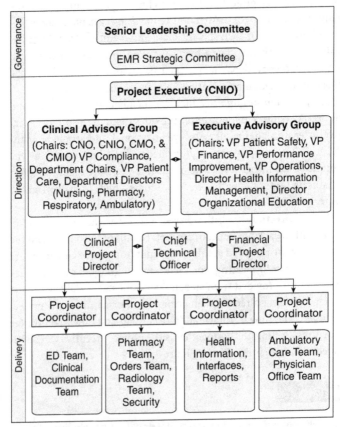

Figure 8.1 Electronic Health Record (EHR) project structure.

CNIO, chief nursing informatics officer; CMIO, chief medical informatics officer; CMO, chief medical officer; CNO, chief nursing officer; EMR, electronic medical record; VP, vice president.

Education and Certifications

The focus of the DNP degree for the CNIO is to provide strategic vision for informatics within the organization. At the DNP level, there are many opportunities for an executive. The capstone project should directly relate to the administrative focus highlighting advocacy and policy. The CNIO at the DNP level assures quality and safety across the organization. This is accomplished through standardization, compliance, accuracy, financial information, and a seamless transition to automation.

Certifications appropriate for the CNIO include the American Nurses Credentialing Center (ANCC, n.d.) and American Organization for Nursing Leadership (AONL, n.d.). The ANCC offers Informatics Nursing Certification (RN-BC) and Nurse Executive, Advanced Certification (NEA-BC). These certifications require minimum hours for clinical practice in the specialty and hours for continuing education in the specialty (ANCC, n.d.). The AONL offers certification as executive nursing practice (CENP). This certification prepares the nurse executive in communication, knowledge, professionalism, and business skills (AONL, n.d.).

The CNIO should be prepared to assist departments, both clinical and financial, in system implementation, assuring that the system is congruent with current operations. The CNIO will oversee system selection process and conduct research as related to informatics and technology. The role will provide direction for the implementation teams and make recommendations for changes as appropriate.

The CNIO will review clinical and business metrics and utilize performance improvement methodologies to implement change. The CNIO will provide the strategic direction for the organization as it relates to informatics and technology.

Challenges and Opportunities

Fast Facts

The most difficult challenge for the DNP-CNIO is to effectively manage change throughout the organization. Understanding change management theory and the implications of change is essential for

(continued)

(continued)

the CNIO. The DNP-CNIO must be able to manage expectations and be realistic in what can be accomplished with implementations. As standardization is realized, there will be pushback from departmental directors and staff. Each will have a unique perspective on what is essential in a clinical information system. However, goals must be met to ensure the vision is accomplished.

There are many opportunities for the DNP-CNIO. Nurses at the administrative level can easily function in this role. One key factor is the DNP-CNIO has the clinical perspective with a background in technology, which allows for a smooth transition. Again, the primary focus is to ensure that the patient remains the center of any informatics change.

DNP Informatics Specialist as Educator

Technology Informatics Guiding Education Reform Initiative

Since the introduction of computers into the workplace for healthcare, there has been an overwhelming need for educators to guide their use. In order to improve nursing practice, education and patient care technology is incorporated into the curriculum and workflow of nurses. The Technology Informatics Guiding Education Reform (TIGER) initiative was developed with a focus on education, community development, and global workforce development (Health Information and Management Systems Society [HIMSS], n.d.-b). This initiative serves as a guide for the DNP informatics specialist educators. There are several TIGER initiatives, recommendations, action steps, and reports available for the informatics nurse educator.

The "Evidence and Informatics Transforming Nursing: developed a 3-year Action Steps towards a 10-year Vision" (HIMSS, 2007). Seven pillars were identified including management and leadership, education, communication and collaboration, informatics design, IT, policy, and culture. The group stressed the need to teach students at the onset of their education. The focus should be on data and practice with informatics providing patient- and evidence-based delivery.

Several academic programs have merged telehealth, electronic forms, decision support, and handheld devices into their curriculum. Recommendations for academic institutions include: adopting informatics competencies in all levels of nursing education; faculty participating in developing programs in informatics; developing a task force to integrate informatics throughout the curriculum; encouraging regulatory bodies to expand support for informatics; measuring informatics knowledge in both educators and students; collaborating with vendors and partners to adopt technology; and recruiting, retaining, and training nurses in the areas of informatics education practice and research (HIMSS, 2007).

TIGER also has a vision for leadership. A collaborative report was developed for nursing executives. The leadership development collaborative team engages leaders from practice and educational settings to develop strategies related to health IT. Several nurse executive health IT activities were identified in this report. There should be leadership development programs including academic graduate programs for nursing informatics and nurse executives; nurse leaders should assess the capabilities of their workforce and address any gaps in terms of health IT; and nurse executives must have an expanded knowledge of budget, regulatory, safety, and security policies related to EHRs (HIMSS, 2010). Identification of core computer competencies is essential for the educator. Nurses in many different roles are required to master technology and incorporate legal and ethical components into the workflow. The DNP informatics specialist educator assists the beginner and novice nurse as they document care, manage patients, and participate in technology initiatives.

Education Programs

One key responsibility for the DNP informatics specialist educator is the planning and execution of an educational program prior to the implementation of a clinical system. The skills required for this include the following:

- Budgeting
- Project management
- Curriculum development
- Validation of end-user competence

Table 8.1

Estimated Cost to Educate Nurses and Other Healthcare Providers in a Large Acute Care Organization

Role	Total Number	Avg Salary	Class Time (hours)	Total Cost (straight time)	Total Cost (overtime)
RN (Med/Surg)	1,000	$50.00	32	$1,600,000.00	$2,400,000.00
RN (ICU/L&D/ED)	400	$50.00	40	$800,000.00	$1,200,000.00
NM/Educator	139	$55.00	32	$244,640.00	$366,960.00
LPN	10	$31.00	24	$7,440.00	$11,160.00
Care Assistant	369	$20.00	12	$88,560.00	$132,840.00
Clerk	329	$21.00	12	$82,908.00	$124,362.00
Tech	158	$23.00	12	$43,608.00	$65,412.00
Totals	2,405			$2,867,156.00	$4,300,734.00

L&D, labor and delivery; LM, licensed midwife; LPN, licensed practical nurse; NM, nurse manager; RN, registered nurse.

In addition, the educator must provide support after the implementation to facilitate a smooth transition to the new clinical system. Knowledge of budgeting is essential. Classes are generally conducted over 1 to 5 days. While the nurses are educated, care will continue seamlessly on their units. The DNP educator must estimate class time and replacement time (Table 8.1). This is a significant investment based upon straight time for class attendees and overtime for replacements. The DNP informatics specialist educator will provide the justification for the high cost, stressing the quality of education and safety on the units.

Training: Another important task is the development of a project plan for training. Key milestones should be identified. The organization should have an existing learning management system. A team is identified for training. The trainers should have skills, which include knowledge of the system, prior experience as a trainer, clinical experience, and ability to communicate effectively and work well with others. The DNP informatics specialist educator will work with human resources to determine the number of end users to be trained. The length of training depends upon the applications to be implemented. Together with the vendor, the DNP educator will identify class duration. For example, medical/surgical nurses generally require the basic education on documentation, medication management, and plan of care. Specialty nurses such as labor and delivery, oncology, emergency room, and intensive care unit require additional education. The process for downloading data from monitors and documenting information on more complex patients accounts for the additional education. Very often, third-party systems must be integrated into the clinical information system. These include cardiac monitoring, fetal monitoring, and triage information.

An *education governance committee* should be identified. The DNP informatics specialist educator should be the chair of this committee. Medical, nursing, and pharmacy educators should be on the committee. In addition, representatives from the staffs of nursing, pharmacists, respiratory therapy, and IT should be committee members. The focus is on inter-professional education. This was defined by the World Health Organization (Hopkins, 2010) as students from different professions educated together to learn about, from, and with each other. This enables effective collaboration and helps to improve health outcomes (Hopkins, 2010).

The committee should oversee the education of the interprofessional staff. This will be done over five phases that will incorporate planning the education to completion and postlive maintenance (Figure 8.2). The first phase includes development of the education plan, methodology, and logistics including setting up a training database. The second phase should be dedicated to curriculum and trainers. As noted, incorporation of policy and procedures into the curriculum is essential. Phase three requires testing the training system and identifying reports and metrics. Phase four finalizes the curriculum, develops competency assessments, skills validation, and detailed education sessions. Phase five occurs after go-live of the clinical information system. At this point, the education governance

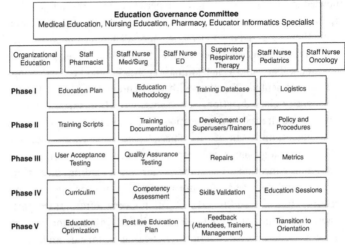

Figure 8.2 Education Governance Committee: The Five Phases of Education.

committee will optimize the educational process; develop a plan for postlive education; and disseminate feedback from attendees, trainers, and management. The last step is a transition into the existing orientation curriculum so that all new hires are educated on the clinical system.

Curriculum development is the responsibility of the DNP informatics specialist educator in collaboration with the vendor and clinical staff. It is necessary to incorporate organizational policy and procedure into class content. This is done in collaboration with the management and nursing education. Nurses are also educated on the workflow changes that will occur with the implementation. Case studies are developed and should relate to the specific patient population for each role.

The scheduling of end users for class can be a difficult task. The learning management system should include the ability for scheduling. It should be an intuitive process allowing managers to schedule their staff based on role-specific educational requirements, the needs of unit staffing, and date and shift employee preference.

The DNP informatics nurse educator ensures that education modules provide the clinical staff with the information necessary to safely provide care to patients. The educator validates training materials for the safety component and ensures competency is achieved prior to granting access to the clinical system. The type of training is determined. This includes computer-based training or in-class lectures. It is also necessary to evaluate computer skills. This is done through an assessment of computer skills and educational needs. The educator will ensure that computer skills are validated and performance is monitored postimplementation.

The vendor should have a separate and distinct training platform within the clinical system. This will allow the DNP informatics specialist educator to populate the training system with patients, orders, and scenarios related to the curriculum. In collaboration with IT, facilities are identified and set up for end-user training.

Curriculum Development in Academia

The DNP informatics specialist as an educator in academia requires a different skill set and role. One aspect is incorporating informatics competencies into the core curriculum for nursing students at all levels of practice. At the baccalaureate level, nurses must have a basic understanding of the management of information and computer technology (Staggers, Gasser, & Cochrane, 2002). Incorporating EHRs and medication management into the clinical experience is essential. The students must be able to use handheld devices, access patient information, and document in a timely manner. The proper use of social media in the workplace must also be addressed. The use of a virtual learning environment can easily facilitate the transition for student nurses to the clinical practice area.

At the graduate level, advanced skills are required. Nursing students must be able to use technology to support patient outcomes. Judgment should be made on trends and patterns from data entered and accessed through the clinical system (Staggers et al., 2002). Academic institutions now offer a master's in nursing informatics. The curriculum for these courses includes the following:

1. Nursing informatics theory
2. Computer science theory
3. Science theory
4. Project management
5. Change management
6. Communication theory

Fast Facts

At the doctoral level, the informatics educator leads in the advancement of research healthcare policy and knowledge management. The Essentials of Doctoral Education for advanced nursing practice include the use of information, IT, and patient care technology to evaluate and resolve ethical and legal issues (American Association of Colleges of Nursing, 2006).

Education and Certifications

The focus of the DNP practice degree for the educator in the informatics specialist role should be on informatics education in both academia and healthcare. At the DNP level, there are many opportunities for an educational focus. The capstone project should directly relate to the education of students or staff. The informatics component of the education should be threaded through each of the courses offered at the DNP level.

Certifications appropriate for the informatics specialist as educator include those from both ANCC and AONL. The ANCC (n.d.) offers informatics nurse certification, nursing professional development certification, and nurse executive certification. These certifications require minimum hours for clinical practice in the specialty and hours for continuing education in the specialty. The AONL (n.d.) offers CENP. This certification prepares the nurse executive to be competent in communication, knowledge, professionalism, and business skills.

The DNP informatics educator should be prepared to design clinical information systems, educate end users, and assess competency post education. The DNP educator should develop performance improvement plans relating to clinical information systems to assure the correct use of the system; in addition, a thorough review of current organizational policy and procedure should be completed. Prior to implementation, new or revised policy should be integrated.

In the classroom, the DNP educator should ensure that informatics skills are seamlessly integrated into the curriculum at all levels. Basic informatics competencies should be met by graduating students. Virtual laboratories and simulation laboratories should be utilized to the fullest potential to ensure students competently use technology to provide patient care.

Challenges and Opportunities

Several challenges exist for the informatics specialist in the educator role. One organizational issue identified is the need to merge past practice among disciplines (Husting & Cintron, 2003). Incorporating student documentation into the curriculum and into clinical practice remains an issue. Lessons learned from computer training can be as simple as allowing the student to practice on new hardware. The trainer must be flexible in both methods and approach. Translating computer terminology for clinical staff is also a challenge. Being able to appropriately time computer training is especially difficult when there are a large number of attendees. For classes that carry over 2 to 4 days, this timing can be daunting. It is important to remember that education must occur as close as possible to the system implementation date. A very significant challenge is the training budget. This must be incorporated into the overall project plan and is as crucial as the cost for devices and the software.

Opportunities for the informatics nurse educator are substantial. Vendors require clinicians and educators to assist their clients. Clinical facilities currently have many full-time employees in this role. Academic institutions utilize the DNP informatics specialist educator both for informatics programs and informatics courses at all levels. This offers a unique opportunity to incorporate nursing science, informatics science, and computer science into the design and education. EHRs are ubiquitous and constantly changing. Being able to participate in this new and exciting field is one of the most rewarding aspects for the educator.

Challenges in academia include budgetary restrictions for virtual and simulated laboratories. Attracting qualified faculty to academic institutions is also a challenge. There is a great demand for informatics nurse specialists in healthcare so that universities must compete for these individuals.

The opportunities in academia include participating in cutting-edge educational technology across all levels. Preparing new nurses for the real world of clinical practice and simulation labs and with the technology available is extremely rewarding.

DNP Informatics Specialist as Project Director

According to the Project Management Institute (PMI) (2009), a *project* is "a temporary endeavor undertaken to create a unique product, service or result" (p. 5). The DNP project director is both a clinical and IT expert who applies best practice to project implementation. In collaboration with the CNIO, the DNP project director manages special projects within the organization. This role requires conducting research related to project management and utilizing performance improvement methodologies within each project. The DNP project manager has specific knowledge of databases and software for programs that support implementations, education, and performance improvement.

The project management framework utilized by the DNP (PMI, 2009) includes tasks such as identifying requirements for projects, establishing clear and achievable objectives, and utilizing ethical and professional conduct within project management. It is essential that the director balances quality, project scope, timelines, and cost. The DNP must be flexible and be able to address the concerns and expectations of the stakeholders. Stakeholders include customers and end users, team members, sponsors, and both positive and negative influencers (PMI, 2009). The project director also utilizes the information management framework within project management. This framework comprises computer skills, informatics knowledge, and informatics skills. They are aligned with informatics competencies and human information-processing skills to result in information management competencies (Staggers et al., 2002).

There are many skills that are necessary for the DNP project director. Those skills include the following:

1. Communication
2. Conflict resolution
3. Flexibility
4. Organizational effectiveness
5. Professionalism
6. Trustworthiness and teamwork (Maciver, 2012).

The DNP must identify how each of the projects under his or her direction contributes to the mission, vision, and values. Each project has an effect on patient safety along with financial implications.

The DNP project director applies sound financial management principles by utilizing budgets and resources appropriately (Lang, 2007). According to the American Association of Colleges of Nursing (2006), the DNP should be prepared to "[e]valuate consumer health information sources for accuracy, timeliness, and appropriateness" (p. 13). The DNP should also be proficient in the use of technology for quality performance and practice through administrative decision-making.

As a project director, there are essential project management skills that are necessary. According to Houston (2012), these skills include analytical thinking, decision-making, organization, motivation, flexibility, effective communication, leadership, facilitation, time management, collaboration, negotiation, and interpersonal skills (p. 19). These skills are not very different from those necessary to give care at the bedside. In the case of the project director, the outcomes are project-specific rather than patient-specific. The project director must ensure that critical success factors are met. These success factors include budget, scope, schedule, teamwork, and communications (Collegiate Project Services, 2009). Signs that your project may be in trouble include not having a clear budget, not having a formal scope plan, ineffective communication, and lack of teamwork (Collegiate Project Services, 2009).

The DNP must stay current with technology to ensure project success. This includes the use of mobile technology and handheld devices utilized in system implementations; these devices include barcode medication administration, smart phones or tablets at the bedside, real-time transmission of data from cardiac monitors, and devices to communicate with other caregivers (Mitchell, 2015). The project director in collaboration with IT evaluates and selects appropriate hardware for system implementations. Again, budgeting is a key component of this selection. The devices must be efficient, secure, and intuitive to use.

The DNP project director is responsible for the change management process. This should be incorporated into each step of the project plan. It includes communication and change management theory. The project director also utilizes project management tools to ensure that milestones are identified and met within each project. One tool that can be used effectively is Microsoft Project. This tool easily documents every step of the project and automatically updates when changes are made to durations or end dates. Other tools are available as well, and many are effective in facilitating documentation of tasks.

The project plan is detailed including such information as project task, duration, start date, and end date. It is essential that certain project tasks are identified as milestones. These milestones are those tasks that must be met at the specific end date to ensure completion of the project at this specific date identified. The milestones are the ones reviewed by senior leadership to ensure that the project is on time. Specific details of each task are reviewed by the project director and coordinators. It is the responsibility of the director to ensure that team members are completing each task on time so that the project is not adversely impacted.

The project director oversees the project management office (PMO) that ensures clinical and business objectives are integrated with technology projects (Isola, Polikaitis, & Laureto, 2006). Some of the functions of the PMO include developing strategic plans for IT, implementing changes, standardizing and using tools in project management, and collaborating with interdisciplinary departments. The overall result should be managing an IT portfolio in collaboration with stakeholders (Isola et al., 2006).

Education and Certifications

Fast Facts

The focus of the DNP degree for the project director is to identify requirements, quality, scope, and budget of an organizational project. The project director ensures that strategic vision for informatics within the organization is threaded through the project plan. At the DNP level, there are many opportunities for a project focus. The capstone project should directly relate and includes the identification of an informatics project to be implemented. The capstone should include a detailed project plan identifying tasks, milestones, budget, scope, and quality. The project director at the DNP level assures quality and safety across the organization during and after project completion. This is accomplished through standardization, compliance, and accuracy.

Certifications appropriate for the project director include those from the ANCC, HIMSS, and PMI. The ANCC offers Informatics Nursing Certification (RN-BC). Certification as a Project Management Professional (PMP)® validates competence to perform in the role of a project manager. This competence includes leading and directing projects and teams. Portfolio Management Professional (PMP)® recognizes advanced experience and skill of portfolio managers. Both are offered by the PMI (n.d.). CPHIMS Certification is a professional certification program for experienced healthcare information and management systems professionals (HIMSS, n.d.-a). Individuals with CPHIMS credential demonstrate a standard of professional knowledge and competence in healthcare information management systems. This certification is offered by HIMSS.

The project director should be prepared to develop, implement, and complete the project plan. This includes meeting milestones, remaining within budget, identifying scope, and transitioning to maintenance. The project director oversees the PMO and all resources associated with the project. Resources include staff responsible for the project such as analysts, super users, stakeholders, and clinical staff. Additional resources include programs and hardware necessary for completion of the project. The project director works in collaboration with the CNIO and the educator to ensure all components of the project are complete.

CONCLUSION

Challenges and Opportunities

Several challenges exist for the project director. The project director must ensure that all disciplines are aligned with the goal of the project. Ensuring that effective communication and change management techniques are in place is crucial for the success of the project. A detailed understanding of the budgetary process is necessary. Flexibility and adaptability are also key components in this role. The project director must be able to adjust to outside influences so that the project remains on time and within budget. Coordinating each phase and each task of the project remains the responsibility of the project director.

Opportunities for the project director are substantial. Both vendors and clinical facilities require staff with these skills. There are a wide range of projects available, so it is easy to find something within the specialty of the project director. Certifications are an excellent way to prepare the project director for this role. Being intimately involved with a project allows the director to ensure patient care outcomes are met and safety is ensured.

REFLECTION QUESTIONS

1. What are the key components for the DNP informatics nurse to be successful?
2. How has nursing informatics evolved over the years?
3. How have these changes in nursing informatics impacted nursing and patient care?
4. How will nursing informatics change your practice as a DNP-prepared nurse?
5. What changes related to informatics have you experienced? Reflect on positive or negative experiences. What could have been done better?
6. How can the informatics field create change in the clinical-focused DNP nurse?
7. What do you believe are the major challenges for your current DNP informatics nurse?
8. How would you plan to implement a major informatics change as a DNP-prepared nurse?

References

American Association of Colleges of Nursing. (2006). *The essentials of doctoral education for advanced nursing practice.* Retrieved from https://www.aacnnursing.org/Portals/42/Publications/DNPEssentials.pdf

American Nurses Association. (2015). *Nursing informatics: Scope and standards of practice* (2nd ed.). Silver Spring, MD: American Nurses Association.

American Nurses Credentialing Center. (n.d.). *Our certifications.* Retrieved from https://www.nursingworld.org/our-certifications

American Organization of Nurse Executives. (2012). *Position paper: Nursing informatics executive leader.* Retrieved from https://www.aonl.org/sites/default/files/aone/informatics-executive-leader.pdf

American Organization for Nursing Leadership. (n.d.). *CENP essentials review course.* Retrieved from https://www.aonl.org/education/cenp-review

Collegiate Project Services. (2009). *Is your project in trouble?* Retrieved from https://s3.amazonaws.com/rdcms-himss/files/production/public/HIMSSorg/Content/files/Code%2087_Is%20Your%20Project%20in%20Trouble_Collegiate%20Services.pdf

Hassett, M. (2006). Case study: Factors in defining the nurse informatics specialists role. *Journal of Healthcare Information Management, 20,* 30–35. Retrieved from https://s3.amazonaws.com/rdcms-himss/files/production/public/HIMSSorg/Content/files/Code%2019%20Case%20Study%20Factors%20in%20Defining%20the%20Nurse%20Informatics%20Specialist%20Role.pdf

Health Information and Management Systems Society. (n.d.-a). *Health information and technology certifications.* Retrieved from https://www.himss.org/health-it-certification

Health Information and Management Systems Society. (n.d.-b). *The TIGER initiative (technology informatics guiding education reform).* Retrieved from https://www.himss.org/professionaldevelopment/tiger-initiative

Health Information and Management Systems Society. (2007). *TIGER initiative: Evidence and informatics transforming education: A 3-year action steps toward a 10-year vision.* Retrieved from https://www.himss.org/library/evidence-and-informatics-transforming-nursing-3-year-action-steps-toward-10-year-vision

Health Information and Management Systems Society. (2010). *TIGER initiative: Revolutionary leadership driving healthcare innovation: The TIGER leadership development collaborative report.* Retrieved from https://www.himss.org/professionaldevelopment/tiger-initiative

Hopkins, D. (Ed.). (2010). *Framework for action on interpersonal education and collaborative practice.* Geneva, Switzerland: World Health Organization Press.

Houston, S. (2012). Nursing's role in IT projects. *Nursing Management, 43,* 18–19. doi:10.1097/01.NUMA.0000409931.77213.40

Husting, P., & Cintron, L. (2003). Healthcare information systems: Education lessons learned. *Journal for Nurses in Staff Development, 19,* 249–253. Retrieved from https://journals.lww.com/jnsdonline/Abstract/2003/09000/HEALTHCARE_INFORMATION_SYSTEMS__EDUCATION_LESSONS.8.aspx

Isola, M., Polikaitis, A., & Laureto, R. (2006). Implementation of a Project Management Office (PMO): Experiences from year 1. *Journal of Healthcare Information Management, 20*, 79–87.

Lang, R. (2007). Project leadership: Key elements and critical success factors for IT project managers. *Journal of Healthcare Information Management, 21*, 2–4.

Maciver, L. (2012). 12 essential soft skills for project managers. *Ezine Articles.* Retrieved from https://ezinearticles.com/?12-Essential-Soft-Skills-for-Project-Managers&id=5935196

Mitchell, M. B. (2015). We save lived: An informatics perspective on innovation. *Nursing, 45*, 20–21. doi:10.1097/01.NURSE.0000459593.78396.c4

Project Management Institute. (n.d.). *Certifications.* Retrieved from https://www.pmi.org/certifications

Project Management Institute. (2009). *A guide to the project management body of knowledge: (PMBOK® Guide)* (4th ed.). Newtown Square, PA: Author.

Staggers, N., Gassert, C., & Curran, C. (2002). A Delphi study to determine informatics competencies for nurses at four levels of practice. *Nursing Research, 51*, 383–390. Retrieved from https://www.nursingcenter.com/journalarticle?Article_ID=286665&Journal_ID=54027&Issue_ID=286655

Further Reading

Anderson, C., & Sensmeier, J. (2014). Nursing informatics: A specialty on the rise. *Nursing Management, 45*, 16–183p. doi:10.1097/01.NUMA.0000449768.37489.ac

Health Information and Management Systems Society. (2018). *2018 HIMSS U.S. leadership and workforce survey.* Retrieved from https://www.himss.org/2018-himss-leadership-and-workforce-survey

Office of the National Coordinator for Health Information Technology. (2019). *Transition issues.* Retrieved from https://www.healthit.gov/sites/default/files/playbook/pdf/ehr-contract-guide-chapter-9.pdf

9

The DNP-Prepared Nurse as an Entrepreneur

"So never lose an opportunity of urging a practical beginning, however small, for it is wonderful how often in such matters the mustard-seed germinates and roots itself."—Florence Nightingale

INTRODUCTION

The Meaning of *Entrepreneur*

The word *entrepreneur* is derived from the French word *entrependre*, which means "to undertake" ("Entrepreneur," n.d.) It has been in use since the mid-1700s, long before nursing as a profession had its beginning. The word *entrepreneur* has evolved over time to mean someone who starts and maintains his or her own business. It also has the connotation that the person who is an entrepreneur is a risk-taker, ambitious, and goes after a dream or vision.

Another word we need to define that is often found in the literature side by side with entrepreneure is "intrapreneur." An *intrapreneur* is someone who has all of the qualities of an entrepreneur but who uses them within an already established corporate environment or business. People with these characteristics are now often given titles like innovation executive or chief innovation officer to denote their role in developing new aspects of the business or new ways of positioning the business. When used in nursing literature, it is not restricted to corporate executives but can be associated with frontline nurses who develop new, creative ways of tackling a problem. Nurses' ideas, born from their problem-solving skills, have long been the impetus and foundation for organizational changes in the institutions where they work. It has been noted however that oftentimes, nurses' contributions to the challenges and ensuing solutions or ideas for change go unnoticed or are undervalued or ignored (Knoff, 2019). While intrapreneurship is alive and well in nursing, this chapter focuses on nurse entrepreneurs who strike out on their own and make their own path in the world of business.

THE EVOLUTION OF THE NURSE AS ENTREPRENEUR

The concept of a nurse entrepreneur may "feel" or sound like a new direction for nurses to explore as a viable career path. Yet it is not. Our nursing history is riddled with and was in fact founded by an entrepreneur—Florence Nightingale herself! Ms. Nightingale was not only the first nurse, the founder of modern nursing, but she was the first nurse entrepreneur. Who would not characterize her a "go-getter" or a person who did not accept risks? She used her talents to create something new. She defined and developed an entirely new profession!

She improved the outcomes of the soldiers wounded in the Crimean war with her "radical" ideas of nutrition, sanitation, and rest; she started the first nursing school; she wrote notes in simple language so that all could understand what her plan was; and she used statistics to give credence to her interventions. Florence Nightingale made these strides from the mid-1800s to the early 1900s and was not the last of the nurse entrepreneurs.

Fast Facts

Other nurse innovators/risk takers/entrepreneurs include Sister Jean Ward who noted vast improvements in babies with jaundice when they were taken out in the sunlight; Lillian Wald who is credited with the founding of the Henry Street Settlement, the precursor to the modern day New York Visiting Nurse Service; Clara Barton the founder of the American Red Cross; and nurses who cared for AIDS patients early in the epidemic who are credited with the development of early care standards for the care provided to these patients with a newly identified disease.

NURSES MAKING HISTORY

Another time that is historically important for entrepreneurial nurses was the turn of the 20th century. During this time, most nurses, up to 80% of all licensed nurses, were employed as independent contractors (Whelan, 2012). Nurses at that time contracted independently with patients and/or families when there was an illness to care for them in their homes. A nurse would work as a private-duty nurse for the duration of the illness, 24 hours a day 7 days a week. When the patient felt better, or died, they were then free to find and accept another position. Nurses made their own schedule, took patients when they wanted, or could, and were completely in control of their work. This was prior to the advent of hospitals as the primary place where people received healthcare.

The next step in entrepreneurism for nurses was the development of nursing registries owned in many cases by nurses. A registry acted as a "middle-woman" who would get the referral from families or physicians and then contact individual nurses to accept or decline the case. As hospitals began burgeoning and replacing home as the primary setting for the delivery of healthcare, nurse registries began to move toward providing care to hospitalized patients. As this change was occurring, some of the registries were owned by the hospital, while some remained under the ownership of nurses (Whelan, 2012). Today's job market does not offer private-duty nursing to the extent that it was seen in the early to mid-20th century. What we do see is the development of travel nurse organizations or home care agencies to supplement staffing and care post-hospitalization. These can also be nurse owned but are more often than not owned by hospital systems or other corporations including groups of physicians.

THE DNP-PREPARED NURSE AS ENTREPRENEUR

As we move forward in nursing and as the healthcare system continues to change at an enormous rate, this is a perfect time to fully embrace our entrepreneurial roots and begin to move more nurses into the role of nurse entrepreneur. The Institute of Medicine report *The Future of Nursing: Leading the Change, Advancing Health* (Committee on the Robert Wood Johnson Foundation Initiative on the Future of Nursing, 2011) is our call to arms for innovation and entrepreneurialism. We need to be creative and think critically and outside the box in order to address and positively affect patient outcomes. And we must claim them as our own and not give up ownership to others.

Nurse entrepreneurship allows nurses to explore their professional potential and independent nursing functions, which impact patient care and outcomes. Entrepreneurship allows nurses to focus on what they value professionally rather than being forced to focus on corporate goals and agendas that may or may not reflect their vision (Wall, 2013). It is often this discontent with the status quo or the changing of the acute care environment to one governed by costs and profits rather than care and compassion that draws nurses to open their own businesses (Wall, 2013).

Nurses who choose entrepreneurial roles are similar to individuals from other professions in terms of some traits that have been identified as being present in these individuals. People who are entrepreneurs often have an internal locus of control, high self-esteem, are risk-takers with a high tolerance for the unknown, have a high need for personal achievement, and are innovative (Dehghanzadeh et al., 2016). Nurses who are entrepreneurs report feelings of empowerment, more positive and meaningful work, greater feelings of fulfillment, increased autonomy, and increased control over their work (Vannucci & Weinstein, 2017; Wall, 2014).

Other attributes used to describe nurse entrepreneurs, which support the role, are intellectual, hard-working, ethical, excellent communication and listening skills, versatility, and adaptability (Cardillo, 2019).

Navigating Fee for Services

A question or concern that surfaces on a fairly regular basis in relation to nurse entrepreneurs is that of fees. There are often two areas of concerns voiced by nonnurses and nurses alike. The first is concerning the legality of nurses charging for nursing services. The second has to do with the ethics or congruency of charging for nursing services and the altruistic mission of nursing to provide care (Kirkman, Wilkinson, & Scahill, 2018; Koch, 2016; Muscari, 2004; Rai, 2007). This should not be surprising as nursing is often depicted as a subservient or ancillary profession of medicine. This is more than likely related to imbalance of power in healthcare institutions, the majority of nurses being female, and the public face of nursing in TV and the movies. Few members of the public know the independent functions of nurses and the education we receive. We are often viewed as "helpers."

This problem of charging a fee is compounded by the fact that many of us, at all levels of nursing, are generally uncomfortable with asking for money for our services. We are also often lacking the knowledge and practical experience in establishing our worth monetarily. The first noted concern about legality needs to be addressed first and foremost.

All nurses thinking about opening a business need to contact the Board of Nursing in the state in which they practice to see what laws govern the ability of a nurse to charge for services. They must also assure that they are clear about what is and is not a nursing service in that state as each state has independent practice acts and laws. Problems will certainly arise for anyone who practices outside the parameters set by the state in which they practice. Along with the legality, potential nurse entrepreneurs should also investigate what if any interventions or services will be reimbursed by private insurances, Medicare, and Medicaid.

The next part of this problem is rooted in education or lack thereof. Nowhere in our education are we taught about business or finance. It is not in any curriculum, except perhaps graduate-level curricula in nursing administration or DNP curricula as a broad topic of healthcare economics. Unless an individual nurse has an interest in these topics or knows he or she is going to want to start a business and take elective courses, these subjects are not covered in our education.

The second part of the problem is more about changing perceptions: our own about our monetary worth and the system's and the public's view of us as ancillary. The majority of nurses begin their careers at in-patient facilities where their service is not monetized, as they are "lumped in" with the daily charge for the room and board of a patient's hospital stay. The altruistic notion that nurses should not charge a fee for services they provide because we are a "caring" profession is not one that has any foundation in the entrepreneurial arena. There is no question that other professionals characterized as "helping" professionals such as audiologists, occupational therapists, speech therapists, pharmacists, physicians, child advocates, social workers, psychological therapists, and physical therapists are paid for their services. Why then would nurses not get paid or find it unethical to get paid for their services? We have expertise, knowledge, and a license indicating competence in our field—all of which can and should be monetized. For nurse entrepreneurs, this is something they must learn to understand and be comfortable with as this is now their livelihood.

EDUCATIONAL REQUIREMENTS

You may have noted something different in this chapter thus far— there has been no mention of the DNP-prepared nurse and entrepreneurship. Rather the most general term *nurse* has been used consistently and liberally until this point. This was purposeful, as any level registered nurse with a license may be an entrepreneur and bill for services. This is because it is the license, not the degree, that sets the boundaries of what is and what is not nursing in each state and therefore what can be charged for.

Some insurance companies will reimburse nursing services, and Medicare reimburses some aspects of nursing care. As stated earlier, before striking out on their own, nurse entrepreneurs should ascertain what is open to reimbursement and what is not. One nurse entrepreneur found that when insurance began reimbursing at a lower rate than what her patients were willing to pay out of pocket for her services, they valued it so much (Muscari, 2004).

In this section, however, I am delineating why, we believe, the DNP-prepared nurse is the ideal nurse entrepreneur. The American Association of Colleges of Nursing's (AACN's) *DNP Essentials of Doctoral Education for Advanced Practice* (2006) is reviewed in relation to its applicability to and enhancement of an entrepreneurial venture. Each of the DNP Essentials inform the practice of DNP-prepared nurses. While some roles inhabited by DNP-prepared nurses emphasize one or more of the Essentials, the DNP-prepared nurse entrepreneur must be well versed in all of them in order to have a successful practice/business. A brief review of each Essential as it pertains to the nurse entrepreneur is as follows:

- Essential I: Scientific Underpinnings for Practice: The DNP-prepared nurse entrepreneur must be expert in the provision of care through the utilization of scientific principles of multiple disciplines, which are part and parcel of nursing.
- Essential II: Organizational and Systems Leadership for Quality Improvement and Systems Thinking: The DNP-prepared nurse entrepreneur must be proficient in all aspects of Essential II. The business a nurse entrepreneur develops and grows is "the system" regardless of whether there are other employees or if the workspace is the living room of his or her house. The DNP-prepared nurse must be able to analyze which care delivery system is best suited to his or her practice. Maintain accountability for all aspects of the business, ensure positive communication, utilize business and finance principles, analyze cost-effectiveness, and anticipate and manage ethical issues as they arise. All of these activities are tied to the competencies of this Essential.
- Essential III: Clinical Scholarship and Analytical Methods for Evidence-Based Practice: The DNP-prepared nurse entrepreneur must be able to use and analyze the literature for new approaches to the population or disease entity on which the business is based. She or he must be responsible for knowing and executing best practices and national guidelines. This then assures the clients that they are receiving the highest quality of care through best practices. The DNP-prepared nurse entrepreneur is well versed in collecting and analyzing data and trends to evaluate outcomes, make adjustments, and develop guidelines.
- Essential IV: Information Systems/Technology and Patient Care Technology for the Improvement and Transformation of Health Care: DNP-prepared nurse entrepreneurs exhibit this essential when they use EMR systems that can assist in the collection of data and monitor outcomes for review and quality insurance. They are capable and adept at evaluating health information marketed to the consumer directly in order to reenforce or reteach information for clients as they interface with them.
- Essential V: Health Care Policy for Advocacy in Health Care: DNP-prepared nurse entrepreneurs must be well-versed in

policy issues, especially those directly impacting the business and populations served. As nurse entrepreneurs, the DNP-prepared nurses develop business and patient care policies that are congruent with state and national guidelines. DNP-prepared nurse entrepreneurs are often on the forefront of social justice issues providing services that fill a gap in nursing in traditional healthcare settings.

- Essential VI: Inter-Professional Collaboration for Improving Patient and Population Health Outcomes: DNP-prepared nurse entrepreneurs must effectively communicate and collaborate. Their business, the business of patients, depends on the ability to perform these skills at a very high level to ensure success. Nurse entrepreneurs need to be able to communicate with other healthcare professionals involved with patients in order to assure high quality and holistic care of the patient. Some nurse entrepreneurs may also depend on others for referrals, making interprofessional collaboration integral to the success of their business.

- Essential VII: Clinical Prevention and Population Health for Improving the Nation's Health: DNP-prepared nurse entrepreneurs are often in the community directly interacting with the public as clients. In this capacity, they can have an enormous impact on the prevention of disease through education and support, which is culturally sensitive and delivered in language that is understandable and appropriate to the client. Strong nurse–client relationships will also add to the achievement of the competencies in this Essential. Evaluation of the care provided or information presented, including statistical analysis of the data, can lead to a wealth of information that can then be utilized by multiple groups and the DNP-prepared nurses in their practice or business.

- Essential VIII: Advanced Nursing Practice: A DNP-prepared nurse entrepreneur practices at the highest level of nursing by providing direct and indirect care through the development of therapeutic relationships. This applies to expert-level care or education or other service provided through the business. This is the foundation of many of the businesses developed by nurses in the entrepreneurial role.

Potential for Additional Education

The flow is seamless from the competencies associated with the DNP Essentials (AACN, 2006), which have been the foundation for the DNP-prepared nurse entrepreneur. There are, however, additional educational components that may be necessary, or at least desirable, for a nurse-owned business to be successful. As stated, Essential II speaks to competencies in principles of finance, business, and economics, yet few DNP programs in the US offer these subjects. While some have global courses, they may be more diverse in their application and not terribly helpful in starting up and running a small business. Functional principles and the usage of principles of these disciplines must be learned from assigned projects during the DNP or through additional coursework beyond the degree requirements. This is similar to recommendations that DNP-prepared nurses who aspire to take faculty positions should take additional coursework in educational topics—this was previously discussed. As the need for fluency in economics, business, and finance is directly written into the Essentials, perhaps, as more programs are developed and those already in existence evolve over-time, specific coursework may be added to the curricula of the future. Doing this would also address the potential lack of knowledge on how developing a business plan is essential to the process of starting a business (Arnaert, Mills, Bruno, & Ponzoni, 2018; Boore & Porter, 2011; Johnson & Garvin, 2017; Koch, 2016; Waxman & Massarweh, 2018).

ROLES AND SETTINGS

DNP-prepared nurse entrepreneurs, in fact all nurse entrepreneurs, can operate a business in a variety of settings, in a variety of roles, across the continuum of care: primary, secondary, or tertiary (The Free Library, 2014). Box 9.1 includes a variety of possible roles according to work settings. However, these will be just small samples of the possibilities, as they are endless and only limited by the imagination of the nurse entrepreneur.

BOX 9.1   ROLES AND SETTING FOR THE DNP-PREPARED ENTREPRENEUR

Primary Care:

Advanced practice nurse-owned practice
Family well care clinic
Pediatric well care clinic
Geriatric well care clinic
Women's well health clinic
Doula practice

Health coaching
Mindfulness coaching
Wellness coaching
Childbirth education
Lactation consultant

Secondary Care:

APRN-owned clinics: acute, short-term illnesses, injury, and early disease treatment
Family care clinics
Pediatric clinics
Geriatrics clinics
Women's health clinics
Disease-specific clinics/businesses: diabetes, congestive heart failure, oncology, foot care, wound care, cardiac care, continence care, and others

Tertiary Care:

More of these roles are intrapreneurial. However, there could be external businesses owned by nurse entrepreneurs doing business with hospitals such as educators and equipment sales.

Fast Facts

In addition to examining nurse entrepreneurial possibilities across the care continuum, there are broader areas of interest that can provide nurses business opportunities, including consulting (health policy, nursing management, specialty nursing, education); home health aide service owner; concierge nursing; and patient care consulting

SOCIAL ENTREPRENEURISM

Many of the roles that can be inhabited by nurse entrepreneurs fall under the category of "social entrepreneurism." Social entrepreneurism differs from traditional entrepreneurism in the outcomes for which it strives (Gilliss, 2011; Rai; 2007). It is developing a business that will lead to positive patient outcomes and thereby positively affect the social good. This does not, however, imply that a business that is considered a social entrepreneurial one, by improving the general well-being of people, cannot or should not be profitable (Rai, 2007).

Our shared history gives us many examples of nurse social entrepreneurism: Florence Nightingale, Lillian Wald, Clara Barton, and others. Each in their own right saw problems, found solutions, and did good for the world at large. Another definition of social entrepreneurism includes income generation through solid business principles for the purpose of sustainability and reinvesting to expand the social good (Rai, 2007). A contemporary example of this is a profit-making APRN gerontological practice in a community setting. APRNs provide holistic care to individuals and communities with the ultimate goal being improved outcomes (Caffrey, 2005). Though the literature does not yet specifically address DNP-prepared APRNs, the Essentials discussed earlier should validate the concept of the fit of DNP-prepared nurses in this role.

OPPORTUNITIES AND CHALLENGES

Oftentimes, opportunities are found in the greatest challenges. It is not different for nurse entrepreneurs. Opportunity for the development of a business is frequently found in the areas of healthcare where there are gaps in care or there is frustration with care delivery or the systems involved in delivering high-quality care. DNP-prepared nurses are educated to identify gaps in care and analyze systems for efficiency and best practice. As more DNP-prepared nurses enter the workforce and do what they were educated to do, more and more entrepreneurial opportunities will present themselves for entrepreneurial ventures.

The Affordable Care Act, which emphasizes preventative and primary care, has provided fertile grounds for nurse entrepreneurs to venture out on their own. Some examples of where nurse entrepreneurs can focus their efforts are aesthetics, alternative treatments, occupational health, preventative health, and aging population.

Characteristics of Entrepreneurship

The literature does speak to personal characteristics of nurses who have chosen entrepreneurship and should be considered when thinking about making the move to become a small business-owner nurse (Colichi, Lima, Bonini, & Lima, 2019; Dehghanzadeh et al., 2016). Some of these characteristics include the following:

Creativity	Hardworking
Risk-taker	Problem-solver/solution-seeker
Intellect	Flexibility
Self motivation	Autonomous
Realistic	Excellent communicator
Confident	Personal belief in one's own ability

Barriers to Entrepreneurs

The barriers encountered by nurse entrepreneurs can come from outside the practice/business or they can be relative to the individual starting it (Arnaert et al., 2018; Boore & Porter, 2011; Colichi et al., 2019; Crunk, 2015; Johnson & Garvin, 2017). Having an earned DNP degree may help with some of the external barriers by adding academic validity to the individual's credentials. Having the degree may also help with some of the internal barriers through confidence, coursework, and a change in personal perception about who one is as a professional.

Barriers Related to Outside Influences

- Insufficient business/management skills and knowledge (curricula/education)
- Raising capital funds (Loans are difficult to get for nurse entrepreneurs.)
- Legal/regulatory issues

- Social issues (The public, more used to physicians, does not know what nurses can do.)
- MD-centered model of care
- Need for collaborating physician with fees (some states)
- A no-change culture
- Need to defend practice to other providers and public

Barriers Related to Individuals

- Gender bias
- Practice balance—as the owner, always working
- Ethical issues—altruism versus profit generating
- Role conflict—taking time away from patients to do administrative work
- Insufficient business/management knowledge and skills
- Scope of practice
- Perfectionism
- Financial stability
- Raising capital funds for start-up—knowledge deficit
- Job/career culture—expected to work in an established job/ institution

SUMMARY

The time for nurse entrepreneurship has arrived—it is the here and now. It is an opportunity for nurses to embrace their history while moving forward toward greater independence and self-determination. Nurse entrepreneurship allows nurses to shine on their own, both inside and outside the medical model. A DNP degree can add value to the credentials of a nurse embarking on a journey of independent entrepreneurism. It says to the public, to the world, that this nurse has achieved the highest level of education as clinician. This should add to the success of DNP-prepared nurse entrepreneurs on their journey toward greater practice and financial independence with the ultimate goal of improved health for individuals and populations by closing the gaps, streamlining the systems, and providing expert care. The sky is the limit!

REFLECTION QUESTIONS

1. How does nursing history relate to the current role of nurse entrepreneurs?
2. What are key characteristics of nurses who chose the role of nurse entrepreneur?
3. What are the top three characteristics of a nurse entrepreneur? Why?
4. Is making a profit by charging for nursing services an ethical dilemma for you? Why, or why not?
5. What advantages does a DNP degree provide for those who choose an entrepreneurial path?
6. What are the common barriers to starting an independent nurse practice?
7. Are you personally drawn to the idea of a nurse entrepreneurial role? Why, or why not?

References

American Association of Colleges of Nursing. (2006). *The essentials of doctoral education for advanced nursing practice.* Retrieved from https://www.aacnnursing.org/Portals/42/Publications/DNPEssentials.pdf

Arnaert, A., Mills, J., Bruno, F. S., & Ponzoni, N. (2018). The educational gaps of nurses in entrepreneurial roles: An integrative review. *Journal of Professional Nursing, 34,* 494–501. doi:10.1016/j.profnurs.2018.03.004

Boore, J., & Porter, S. (2011). Education for entrepreneurship in nursing. *Nurse Education Today, 31,* 184–191. doi:10.1016/j.nedt.2010.05.016

Caffrey, R. A. (2005). Community care gerontological nursing: The independent nurse's role. *Journal of Gerontological Nursing, 31,* 18–25. doi:10.3928/0098-9134-20050701-06

Cardillo, D. (2019). Nursing and entrepreneurship: Perfect together. *Nebraska Nurse, 42,* 10–11.

Colichi, R. M. B., Lima, S. G. S., Bonini, A. B. B., & Lima, S. A. M. (2019). Entrepreneurship and nursing: Integrative review. *Revista Brasileira de Enfermagem, 72,* 321–330. doi:10.1590/0034-7167-2018-0498

Committee on the Robert Wood Johnson Foundation Initiative on the Future of Nursing. (2011). *The future of nursing: Leading change, advancing health.* Washington, DC: National Academies Press.

Crunk, C. (2015). Advanced practice ownership: Is it right for you? *Tennessee Nurse, 78*, 10.

Dehghanzadeh, M. R., Kholasehzadeh, G., Birjandi, M., Antikchi, E., Sobhan, M. R., & Neamatzadeh, H. (2016). Entrepreneurship psychological characteristics of nurses. *Acta Medica Iranica, 54*, 595–599. Retrieved from http://acta.tums.ac.ir/index.php/acta/article/view/5162

Entrepreneur. (n.d.). In *Online etymology dictionary*. Retrieved from https://www.etymonline.com/word/entrepreneur

The Free Library. (2014). *An idea whose time has come: nursing entrepreneurialism*. Retrieved from https://www.thefreelibrary.com/An+idea+whose+time+has+come%3a+nursing+entrepreneurialism.-a0408158289

Gilliss, C. L. (2011). The nurse as social entrepreneur: Revisiting our roots and raising our voices. *Nursing Outlook, 59*, 256–257. doi:10.1016/j.outlook.2011.07.003

Johnson, J. E., & Garvin, W. S. (2017). Advanced practice nurses: Developing a business plan for an independent ambulatory clinical practice. *Nursing Economic$, 35*, 126–141. Retrieved from https://www.questia.com/magazine/1P4-1907287050/advanced-practice-nurses-developing-a-business-plan

Kirkman, A., Wilkinson, J., & Scahill, S. (2018). Thinking about health care differently: Nurse practitioners in primary health care as social entrepreneurs. *Journal of Primary Health Care, 10*, 331–337. doi:10.1071/HC18053

Knoff, C. R. (2019). A call for nurses to embrace their innovative spirit. *Online Journal of Issues in Nursing, 24*, 1. doi:10.3912/OJIN.Vol24No01PPT48

Koch, G. (2016). The RN entrepreneur who owns their own business. *Oregon State Board of Nursing Sentinel, 35*, 10–11.

Muscari, E. (2004). Establishing a small business in nursing. *Oncology Nursing Forum, 31*, 177–179. doi:10.1188/04.ONF.177-179

Rai, S. D. (2007). Social entrepreneurship in nursing—A tool for learning, advocacy and income generation. *Singapore Nursing Journal, 34*, 7–13.

Vannucci, M. J., & Weinstein, S. M. (2017). The nurse entrepreneur: Empowerment needs, challenges, and self-care practices. *Nursing: Research and Reviews, 7*, 57–66. doi:10.2147/NRR.S98407

Wall, S. (2013). Nursing entrepreneurship: Motivators, strategies and possibilities for professional advancement and health system change. *Nursing Leadership, 26*, 29–40. doi:10.12927/cjnl.2013.23450

Wall, S. (2014). Self-employed nurses as change agents in healthcare: Strategies, consequences, and possibilities. *Journal of Health Organization & Management, 28*, 511–531. doi:10.1108/JHOM-03-2013-0049

Waxman, K., & Massarweh, L. J. (2018). Talking the talk: Financial skills for nurse leaders. *Nurse Leader, 16*, 101–106. doi:10.1016/j.mnl.2017.12.008

Whelan, J. C. (2012). When the business of nursing was the nursing business: The private duty registry system, 1900–1940. *Online Journal of Issues in Nursing, 17*, 1. doi:10.3912/OJIN.Vol17No02Man06

10

The Power of Change

"Embrace the change, reach your highest potential, and embark on the most rewarding and innovative degree for nursing, the DNP."—Denise Menonna-Quinn DNP, MSN, RN-BC, AOCNS, BMTCN

INTRODUCTION

The Power of Change

Before examining how the power of change can be equated to doctor of nursing practice (DNP)-prepared nurses, we need to understand the meanings of the terms. *Power* itself has numerous meanings, which can be applied to different professional and personal situations. *Power* has several definitions. It can mean the following:

1. Provide an effect
2. Produce legal implications
3. Performing in a specific manner to create an effect
4. Have control of another individual
5. Related to physical movement
6. Related to moral compass
7. Have control in the political arena

These definitions can be theoretically connected to nursing, especially for the DNP-prepared nurse and the numerous roles available within which to practice, such as nurse practitioner, educator, administrator, and entrepreneur. The multiple definitions have the capability to be applicable to the different role options for the DNP career path. For example, political control or influence can be directly related to the DNP Essential V: Healthcare Policy for Advocacy in Health (American Association of Colleges of Nursing [AACN], 2006).

THE INEVITABILITY OF CHANGE

Change is happening on personal, professional, and political levels. Stefancyk, Hancock, and Meadows (2013) described "change in today's healthcare landscape is daily, if not hourly, reality" (p. 13). This quote speaks volumes regarding delivering care in any healthcare setting. However, the beauty of change is that it can offer new and exciting thoughts, clinical processes, and most importantly patient and organizational outcomes.

Change is a complex word and has numerous meanings. Fundamentally, change is related to producing or making a difference. Other terms that can be used to refer to change are as follows:

- Conversion
- Metamorphosis
- Mutations
- Shifts
- Transformation
- Translation
- Transmutation
- Transubstantiation ("Change," n.d.)

Regardless of which term is chosen to describe change, change is the impetus for the current healthcare environment. Change can be considered a friend to the DNP degree and the DNP nurse. For example, the original design of the degree was for the nurse practitioner, not the educator nor administrator; however, with the change of student applicants, in the education and administration roles, numerous opportunities have developed for the DNP-prepared nurse. The changes for nonnurse practitioners pursuing the DNP degree are positive ones. These multiple definitions can assist the DNP-prepared nurse to be successful with changes in practice. It is critical for DNP-prepared nurses to understand the importance of becoming proactive, innovative, and involved with change and the change process.

THE CHANGING HEALTHCARE ENVIRONMENT

Combining power with change is extremely important, especially in the healthcare arena and more specifically nursing. The healthcare environment is experiencing a huge fluctuation in how patient care is delivered. Healthcare professionals, providers, leaders, and organizations need to understand and embrace change in order to meet the demands of the complex and sometimes volatile healthcare climate. Therefore, change needs to be addressed in numerous fashions. Change needs to occur in the following areas in order to assist in making a difference in today's healthcare:

1. Change healthcare professionals' thought processes of how patient care is delivered.
2. Embrace the change in DNP-prepared nurse roles and opportunities.
3. Change the mechanisms of how and where care is delivered.
4. Understand the global awareness of the current healthcare disparities.
5. Work to change the financial issues related to healthcare delivery.

DRIVERS OF CHANGE IN THE HEALTHCARE ENVIRONMENT

The healthcare climate has drastically changed within the past decade. Salmond and Echevamia (2017) identified drivers of change that include the following:

1. Cost
2. Waste
3. Lack of standardization
4. Quality
5. Healthcare infrastructure

6. Mistargeted incentives/reimbursement
7. Aging population
8. Chronic illness
9. Healthcare disparities

There have been major shifts in how healthcare providers practice, deliver care, and bill for services. The roles of who is delivering care to patients and families have also changed. Additionally, the aging population, increased complex invasive and noninvasive treatment options, and numerous pharmaceutical and technological advantages have impacted the changes in healthcare. Following is an outline of important issues related to the changes in healthcare which DNP-prepared nurses can positively impact:

1. Patient access to healthcare
2. Insurance companies' collaborations
   a. Increased costs of healthcare
   b. Managed care programs
   c. Medicare and Medicaid requirements
3. Healthcare model
   a. Focus on preventative healthcare
      i. Wellness
      ii. Vaccines
      iii. Preventive screening measures
   b. Focus related to patient-centered care
      i. Pharmacy connections
      ii. Greater involvement of patient
         1. Access to electronic health records
4. Importance of positive patient outcomes
   a. Eliminate potential for complications
      i. Infections
      ii. Prolonged admissions
      iii. Readmissions
      iv. Patient compliance
5. Financial/billing
   a. No longer fee for service
   b. Development of hospital systems/networks
   c. Less private practices

Fast Facts

Change is imperative to meet the demands of the current health-care challenges/issues. The DNP-prepared nurse has an amazing opportunity to combine forces with legislations, healthcare systems, administrators, and high-level leaders, as well as patients and their families to develop, initiate, and implement solutions.

THE NEED FOR DNP-PREPARED NURSES TO LEAD CHANGE

Nursing is at the forefront of change. Salmond and Echevarria (2017) stated that the shift in healthcare "requires a new or enhanced set of knowledge, skills and attitudes around wellness and population care with a renewed focus on patient-centered care, care coordination, data analytics and quality improvement" (p. 12). The recommendations from these authors align with the DNP Essentials (AACN, 2006). Therefore, the literature is supporting the numerous and highly qualified DNP-prepared nurses to lead change.

DNP-prepared nurses have advanced knowledge, increased clinical skills, and understanding of the importance of the financial aspect of healthcare and are invaluable to organizations and patients within the complex healthcare environment. Newland (2017) elegantly stated that "DNP preparation are making a difference in the quality of care patients receive and the healthcare outcomes they experience" (p. 8).

CHANGE MODELS AND THEORIES

For change to be successful, it requires a well thought out plan and use of a theory/model. This section is designed for the DNP-prepared nurse to have a general overview of the potential change theories that have been previously used in the nursing, leadership, and management literature. An appropriate model/theory needs to be researched and chosen. There is an abundant amount of change theories/models available. Following are a few examples and options of change theories/models that have been identified, discussed, and used in the nursing literature to identify, promote, and implement changes.

It is important to understand that each change theory has its own advantages and disadvantages. The best individual to choose the change theory/model is the change agent. It is the change agent's decision to choose which model would be best for the situation of change. In this chapter, the change agent is the DNP-prepared nurse.

The DNP-prepared nurse must also realize that there are several commonalities of change steps and process between each of the following models/theories:

1. Lewin's change theory
2. Lippitt's change theory
3. Kotter's change theory
4. Rogers's change theory

Lewin's Change Theory

Kurt Lewin was a psychologist who developed the model in the 1950s. His theory/model has been utilized in nursing and organizations to implement practice changes. Shirey (2013) cited Lewin was known as a "pioneer in the study of group dynamics and organizational development" (p. 69). The model consisted of three stages, which are based upon driving forces that are in motion to push and cause an imbalance in equilibrium in order to promote a change to occur. Lewin's steps include unfreezing, change, and refreezing (Petiprin, n.d.; Shirey, 2013; Wojciechowski, Pearsall, Murphy, and French, 2016).

1. Unfreezing
   a. Determine the issue/situation of change
   b. Identification of change agents
      i. DNP-prepared nurses
   c. Development of solutions
   d. Plan change
2. Change
   a. Detailed plan of action
      i. Clear concise communication
   b. Mobilization of key individuals to promote change
   c. Coaching

   d. Brainstorming
   e. Mentoring
3. Refreezing
   a. Establishment of change
   b. Development of new equilibrium
   c. Monitoring success of change

Lippitt's Change Theory

Lippitt derived a seven-step change process that was an expansion of Lewin's change model. In this theory, the focus is on the role and responsivity of the change agent (Kritsonis, 2005; Mitchell, 2013).

Step 1: Diagnose the problem
Step 2: Assess the motivation and capacity for change
Step 3: Assess the change agent motivation and resources
   1. Resources
   2. Power
   3. Stamina
   4. Commitment
Step 4: Define the change process
Step 5: Define the role of the change agent
   1. Facilitator
   2. Cheerleader
   3. Expert
Step 6: Maintain the change
   1. Support
   2. Communication
   3. Feedback
Step 7: Disengage the use of the change agent
   1. Successful implementation of the change within the organization

Several authors have compared the Lippitt's change theory with the nursing process based on assessment, planning, implementation, and evaluation. The DNP-prepared nurse may find the Lippitt's model useful for practice changes due to the ability to be related to the nursing process.

Kotter's Change Theory

Kotter, a professor at the Harvard Business School, developed an eight-step change process in 1995. Spear (2016) identified that "Kotter's model has been criticized because he cited no references and it was solely based on personal experience and research" (p. 60). Other authors have examined Kotter's eight-step model. The literature supports and recognizes that the change theory is popular due to the ease of the steps and usable format. Kotter has moved his focus from research to the development of private business to aid and execute change for leaders and organizations. Nursing is not the only profession that has utilized this change theory. For example, Wheeler and Holmes (2017) performed a study that identified the transformation of two libraries using Kotter's eight-step change model. Kotter's change theory stipulates the following (Henry et al., 2017; Kotter, n.d.; Small et al., 2016; Spear, 2016):

1. Create a sense of urgency
   a. Recognize the problem
   b. Create an opportunity of change
   c. Motivate the key player
2. Build a guiding coalition
   a. Define the key individuals
      i. Managers
      ii. Nurses
      iii. DNP-prepared nurses
3. Form a strategic vision and initiatives
   a. Stress the positive outcomes
   b. Develop a specific plan
4. Communicate vision
   a. Enlist a volunteer army
   b. Develope a team
      i. Clear communication
5. Enable action by removing barriers
   a. Empower key individuals
   b. Eliminate barriers to change
6. Generate short-terms wins
   a. Emphasize the positive aspects of change
   b. Gain momentum for the change

7. Sustain acceleration
    a. Coach and support
    b. Ensure available resources
8. Institute change
    a. Develope new process

Rogers's Change Theory

Rogers's change theory is also identified as the *diffusion of innovation*. This change theory involves a five-step process. The concept of this theory is based upon the communication of the innovation via social groups and organizations. This theory also revolves around the change agent. This model can be a good choice for a DNP-prepared nurse to utilize for a change project. DNP-prepared nurses have the skill set to perform as excellent change agents (Hilz, 2000; Mitchell, 2013).

Stage 1: Knowledge
    1. Be awareness of issue
    2. Educate
    3. Communicate
Stage 2: Persuasion
    1. Determine the interest
    2. Gather information
    3. Educate peer-to-peer
    4. Use champions
        a. Disseminate information of change project/practice
Stage 3: Decision
    1. Accept or reject the change
Stage 4: Implementation
    1. Develop plan for the change
        a. Detail steps
    2. Implement new process
Stage 5: Confirmation
    1. Support the change
    2. Validate the change
    3. Adopt the change

DNP NURSES AS CHANGE AGENTS

Change agents are imperative to nursing and healthcare systems. Lonadier (2016) remarked in an editorial that "change though a constant, rarely happens on its own. Every change whether small or large, requires a person who first had a vision and was willing to spend time working to implement the change. Change agents are the catalysts that help bring about change" (p. 1). This quote clearly recognized the power of change but more importantly identified *who* is responsible for making the change. Change agents are crucial to the change process. DNP-prepared nurses have the potential and ability to evoke change and make an impact on patients, organizations, and global health issues. Therefore, a fundamental question needs to be asked: Are you willing to be the DNP-prepared nurse who will add a significant amount of change to the healthcare environment?

The roles of DNP-prepared nurses are exciting and innovative and can be infused into numerous practice settings and situations. The DNP-prepared nurses are fully equipped to deal with the healthcare challenges and can be a huge asset to reaching the goals of a positive change agent.

Bowie, DeSocio, and Swanson (2019) performed a study of the impact of the DNP degree and the graduate's role and practice. The results revealed "the overarching theme, 'becoming more: re-envisioning self as agent of change'" (p. 280). Sherrod and Goda (2016) elegantly stated "the DNP-prepared leader possesses key traits to serve as a change agent within complex healthcare environments" (p. 15).

These are powerful statements and provide support that the DNP-prepared nurses are major contenders of change within the health climate. The next step is to examine how DNP-prepared nurses can demonstrate to be the *best* change agents. Change agent qualities are essential to lead change. Michigan State University (2019) identified the following effective change agent qualities to demonstrate the following:

1. Flexibility
2. Diverse knowledge
3. Results oriented and focused
4. Ownership and responsibility
5. Active and effective listening skills

In addition to the abovementioned qualities, the literature demonstrated in the organizational journals the characteristics of successful change agents (Box 10.1). Although these qualities have been denoted in the business arena and the change agent is identified as a trainer and/or consultant, the fundamental concepts can be applied to the DNP-prepared nurse.

BOX 10.1   CHARACTERISTICS AND CAPABILITIES OF SUCCESSFUL CHANGE AGENTS

1. Hemophily: the connection and similarity between the change agent and the client/or organization
2. Empathy: the emotional connection between the change agent and client/organization, which can lead to increased communication
3. Linkage: the bond/collaboration between the change agent and client/organization
4. Proximity: the relationship between the change agent and the organization is imperative to the change process
5. Structuring: the development of a well-planned change process
6. Capacity: the importance of the available resources needed for the change
7. Openness: the degree of open environment from both the change agent and the organization to foster respect, trust, and communication
8. Reward: the higher the reward for all beneficiaries, the more inclined the individuals will support the change
9. Energy: related to the amount of mental and physical energy required to obtain the proposed change
10. **Synergy: the word** *synergy* itself means the connection/ interaction between two or more individuals, organizations, or products in order to produce a combined greater effect and is better than individual effects. It's the concept of the whole being greater than the sum of its parts ("Synergy," n.d.). Therefore, meaning the right individuals, resources and actions are implemented and utilized (Imhonopi & Urim, 2011; Prachi, 2015).

These qualities and capabilities can be invaluable to the DNP-prepared nurse as the change agent. The DNP-prepared nurse will have to use the DNP Essentials to recognize, analyze, and implement these characteristics in order to produce a successful change project. Each step will take time, research, analysis, determination, excellent communication, and reading and writing skills to meet the objectives.

Potential Barriers to Change

Just as important as understanding the change process, DNP-prepared nurses need to be astutely aware of the potential barriers. Barriers are dependent on the specific project. The barriers need to be identified and analyzed in order to combat the negative effects to the change process. See Table 10.1 for common reactions to change.

Table 10.1

Common Reactions to Change and Associated Actions to Promote Change	
Common Reactions to Change	**Change Agent Action and Goals to Promote Change**
Denial Individuals continue to use old methods and/or processes	Provide detailed and accurate information regarding the change and change process
Resistance Negative questions, comments, and disregard for change	Active listening Provide empathy Allow opportunities to alleviate anxiety and concerns
Exploration Individuals explore the change process	Involve staff in change process Encourage team support
Commitment Individuals acknowledge and understand the benefits of the change/new practice	Change agent role is complete Provide support Exit the change process Let individuals manage themselves

Source: Data from Management Sciences for Health (2004). Leading changes in practices to improve health. *The Manager, 13*(3), 1–24.

FUTURE DIRECTIONS

As DNP nurses are engaging in new and exciting roles such as leadership, education, and clinical practice, increased studies related to tracking of DNP roles and opportunities need to be performed. Having the ability to quantify the roles will provide invaluable information to academic educators, leaders, organizations, and of course patients. Creating evidence and data of the benefits of DNP-prepared nurses will provide support and solidify the importance of these roles. It is imperative that DNP-prepared nurses take an active role in demonstrating the value of the degree and career opportunities.

The literature is recognizing the importance of DNP-prepared nurses advocating for themselves and determining their worth in the new healthcare environment. The following authors have made these observations:

1. Bowie et al. (2019) concluded that "If employers receive evidence that the DNP degree can positively impact patient outcomes and cost-effectiveness, the value of the DNP prepared advanced practice nurses may be realized and recognized" (p. 284).
2. Tussing et al. (2018) stated that "Nurses prepared at the DNP level must demonstrate their value to healthcare administrators and nurse executives by sharing their outcomes and engaging in empirically based work to substantiate their value."
3. Pritham and White (2016) revealed that "small, independent surveys have made efforts to measure the DNP degrees value, but this has not been done on a wider scale."

Therefore, it would behoove DNP-prepared nurses and organizations to track the following:

1. Number of DNP-prepared nurses in the organization
2. What roles DNP nurses have within the organization
3. Financial benefits of utilizing DNP-prepared nurses in the various roles
4. Monitor outcomes of patients who are seen by DNP nurses
5. Track the number and outcomes of evidence-based practice projects and research initiated or collaborated with DNP-prepared nurses

SUMMARY

Healthcare is in a huge state of flux. Healthcare administrators, physicians, NPs, and nurses of all specialties are grossly impacted; therefore, who better than a DNP-prepared nurse to be at the forefront of change? DNP-prepared nurses are being summoned to the table to examine, evaluate, speak to, and participate in the numerous change projects, including the following:

- Program development
- Evidence-based practice changes
- Research projects
- Cost containment initiatives
- Quality improvement

Fast Facts

DNP-prepared nurses are great candidates to participate in change because they possess the knowledge base of the healthcare environment and understand the importance of positive patient outcomes and the need for cost containment.

Sherrod and Goda (2016) acknowledged the "redesign of healthcare models and delivery systems requires leaders who are prepared at the doctoral level to sustain and lead the change required for us to be successful" (p. 15). The DNP degree has so many positive opportunities, personal and professional. Please join the DNP arena and continue to make outstanding, positive changes for yourself, patients, and organizations.

REFLECTION QUESTIONS

1. How do you define the power of change and its relationship with your current practice?
2. What healthcare issues have led to a change in your current practice? What are the advantages and disadvantages of the change?

(continued)

(*continued*)

3. Which change theory or model would you choose as a DNP-prepared nurse, and why?

4. Reflect on practice changes or projects you have seen in your current practice. Which theory or model was utilized? Did it lead to success or failure?

5. What change qualities and characteristics are the most important to your practice and your future as a DNP-prepared nurse?

6. What are the barriers to change in your current practice? How can a DNP-prepared nurse eliminate these barriers?

7. What outcome measures within your current organization can the DNP-prepared nurse track?

References

American Association of Colleges of Nursing. (2006). *The essentials of doctoral education for advanced nursing practice.* Retrieved from https://www.aacnnursing.org/Portals/42/Publications/DNPEssentials.pdf

Bowie, B., DeSocio, J., & Swanson, K. (2019). The DNP degree: Are we producing the graduates we intended? *The Journal of Nursing Administration, 49,* 280–285. doi:10.1097/NNA.0000000000000751

Change.(n.d.). *Thesaurus.com.* Retrieved from http://www.thesaurus.com/browse/change

Henry, L., Hansson, C., Haughton, V., Waite, A., Bowers, M., Siegrist, V., & Thompson, E. (2017). Application of Kotter's theory of change to achieve baby friendly designation. *Nursing for Women's Health, 21,* 372–382. doi:10.1016/j.nwh.2017.07.007

Hilz, L. (2000). The informatics nurse specialist as change agent: Application of innovation-diffuse theory. *Computers in Nursing, 18,* 272–281.

Imhonopi, D. F., & Urim, U. M. (2011). Organisational change management and worker's behaviour: A critical review. *International Journal of Development and Management Review, 6,* 216–227. Retrieved from https://www.ajol.info/index.php/ijdmr/article/view/66996

Kotter. (n.d.). 8-step process. Retrieved from https://www.kotterinc.com/8-steps-process-for-leading-change

Kritsonis, A. (2005). Comparison of change theories. *International Journal of Scholarly Academic Intellectual Diversity, 8,* 1–7.

Lonadier, R. (2016). Are you a change agent? *National Association of Orthopedic Nurses, 35,* 1–2.

Management Sciences for Health. (2004). Leading changes in practices to improve health. *The Manager, 13*, 1–24.

Michigan State University. (2019). *Qualities of effective change agents*. Retrieved from http://www.michiganstateuniversityonline.com/resources/leadershi/qualities-of-effective-change-agents

Mitchell, G. (2013). Selecting the best theory to implement planned change. *Nursing Management, 20*, 32–37. doi:10.7748/nm2013.04.20.1.32.e1013

Newland, J. (2017). Growth of DNP degree: Promoting change and improving quality care. *The Nurse Practitioner, 44*, 8. doi:10.1097/01.NPR.0000554090.87523.b6

Petiprin, A. (n.d.). Lewin's change theory. Retrieved from http://nursing-theory.org/theories-and-models/lewin-change-theory.php

Prachi, J. (2015). Characteristics and capabilities of successful change agents. *Management Study Guide Content*. Retrieved from http://www.managementstudyguide.com/portal/about-us

Pritham, U., & White, P. (2016). Assessing DNP impact. Using program evaluations to capture healthcare system change. *The Nurse Practitioner, 41*, 44–53. doi:10.1097/01.NPR.0000481509.24736.c8

Salmond, S., & Echevarria, M. (2017). Healthcare transformation and changing roles for nursing. *Orthopedic Nursing, 36*, 12–25. doi:10.1097/NOR.0000000000000308

Sherrod, B., & Goda, T. (2016). DNP-prepared leaders guide healthcare system change. *Nursing Management, 47*, 13–16. doi:10.1097/01.NUMA.0000491133.06473.92.

Shirey, M. (2013). Lewin's theory of planned change as strategic resource. *Journal of Nursing Administration, 43*, 69–72. doi:10.1097/NNA.0b013e31827f20a9

Small, A., Gist, D., Souza, D., Dalton, J., Magny-Normilus, C., & David, D. (2016). Using Kotter's change model for implementing bedside handoff: A quality improvement project. *Journal of Nursing Care/Quality, 31*, 304–309. doi:10.1097/NCQ.0000000000000212

Spear, M. (2016). How to facilitate change. *Plastic Surgical Nursing, 36*, 58–61. doi:10.1097/PSN.0000000000000139

Stefancyk, A., Hancock, B., & Meadows, M. (2013). The nurse manager: Change agent, change coach? *Nursing Administration Quarterly, 37*, 13–17. doi:10.1097/NAQ.0b013e31827514f4

Synergy. (n.d.). In *Merriam-Webster's online dictionary*. Retrieved from https://www.merriam-webster.com/dictionary/synergy

Tussing, T., Brinkman, B., Francis, D., Hixon, B., Labardee, R., & Chipps. E. (2018). The impact of the doctorate of nursing practice nurse in a hospital setting. *Journal of Nursing Administration, 48*, 600–602. doi:10.1097/NNA.0000000000000688

Wheeler, T., & Holmes, K. (2017). Rapid transformation of two libraries using Kotter's eight steps of change. *Journal of the Medical Library Association*, *105*, 276–281. doi:10.5195/jmla.2017.97

Wojciechowski, E., Pearsall, T., Murphy, P., & French, E. (2016). A case review: Integrating Lewin's theory with Lean's system approach for change. *Online Journal of Issues in Nursing*, *21*, 4. doi:10.3912/OJIN .Vol21No02Man04

Further Reading

Beeber, A., Palmer, C., Waldrop, J., Lynn, M., & Jones, C. (2019). The role of doctor of nursing practice: Prepared nurses in practice settings. *Nursing Outlook*, *67*, 354–364. doi:10.1016/j.outlook.2019.02.006

Index

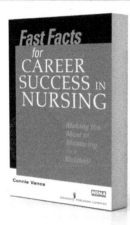
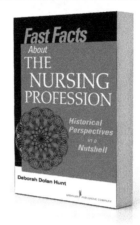
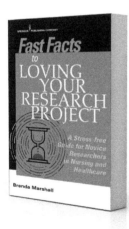
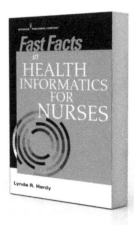